Motivating People to Be Physically Active

Physical Activity Intervention Series

Bess H. Marcus, PhD

Director of Physical Activity Research
Centers for Behavioral and Preventive Medicine
Brown Medical School and The Miriam Hospital

LeighAnn H. Forsyth, PhD

Assistant Professor
of Clinical and Health Psychology
Cleveland State University

Steven Blair, PED

Series Editor
Director of Research
The Cooper Institute

Human Kinetics

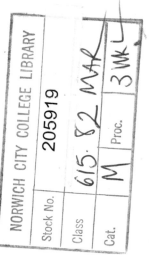

Library of Congress Cataloging-in-Publication Data

Marcus, Bess, 1961-
   Motivating people to be physically active / Bess Marcus,
LeighAnn Forsyth.
      p. ; cm. -- (Physical activity intervention series)
   Includes bibliographical references and index.
   ISBN 0-7360-4064-1 (soft cover : alk. paper)
   1. Exercise therapy. 2. Exercise--Psychological aspects.
3. Motivation (Psychology) 4. Health behavior. 5. Physical edu-
cation and training.   I. Forsyth, LeighAnn, 1967- . II. Title.
III. Series
   [DNLM: 1. Physical Fitness. 2. Exercise. 3. Health Behavior.
4. Motivation. 5. Program Development.   QT 255 M322m
2003]
   RM725.M373 2003
   615.8'2--dc21

2002009228

ISBN: 0-7360-4064-1

Developmental Editor: Renee Thomas Pyrtel; **Assistant Editors:** Amanda S. Ewing, Kim Thoren; **Copyeditor:** Karen Bojda; **Proofreader:** Sarah Wiseman; **Indexer:** Cheryl Landes; **Permission Manager:** Dalene Reeder; **Graphic Designer:** Nancy Rasmus; **Graphic Artist:** Kathleen Boudreau-Fuoss; **Photo Manager:** Leslie A. Woodrum; **Cover Designer:** Keith Blomberg; **Photographer (interior):** Leslie A. Woodrum, unless otherwise noted; **Art Manager:** Kelly Hendren: **Illustrator:** Brian McElwain; **Printer:** United Graphics

Printed in the United States of America   10 9 8 7 6 5 4

Human Kinetics
Web site: www.HumanKinetics.com

United States: Human Kinetics
P.O. Box 5076
Champaign, IL 61825-5076
800-747-4457
e-mail: humank@hkusa.com

Canada: Human Kinetics
475 Devonshire Road, Unit 100
Windsor, ON N8Y 2L5
800-465-7301 (in Canada only)
e-mail: orders@hkcanada.com

Europe: Human Kinetics
107 Bradford Road
Stanningley
Leeds LS28 6AT, United Kingdom
+44 (0)113 255 5665
e-mail: hk@hkeurope.com

Australia: Human Kinetics
57A Price Avenue
Lower Mitcham, South Australia 5062
08 8277 1555
e-mail: liaw@hkaustralia.com

New Zealand: Human Kinetics
Division of Sports Distributors NZ Ltd.
P.O. Box 300 266 Albany
North Shore City, Auckland
0064 9 448 1207
e-mail: blairc@hknewz.com

To my husband, Dan,
for his constant love and support;
to my awesome kids, Brittany and Josh,
who make each day exciting and special;
to my mom, Betty, for always believing in me;
to my late father, Ben, for teaching me
to have faith in the change process;
to my exercise buddies,
Nancy, Michelle, Kristin, and Joan,
who help me keep everything in perspective.

BHM

To my husband, Paul,
for sticking with me through the craziness;
my kids, Olivia and Evan,
who never fail to bring me perspective;
my loving parents, James and Wilma Hock,
who inspire me;
and the Mom's Club members,
Natalie, Jane, Liz, and Lauren,
who share my laughter and tears
when I need it the most.

LAF

CONTENTS

v

Part II Applications

Conclusive evidence confirms the hazards of a sedentary lifestyle and the health benefits of regular physical activity. In the last 10 years, reports by the U.S. Surgeon General, the Centers for Disease Control and Prevention, the American College of Sports Medicine, the National Institutes of Health, and the American Heart Association have identified physical inactivity as a major public health problem. The culmination of discussions from these expert groups led to the revolutionary public health recommendation: "Sedentary adults should accumulate at least 30 minutes of moderate-intensity physical activity over the course of most, preferably all, days of the week."

Another recent development is the emergence of physical activity intervention research that focuses on the application of psychological theories and behavioral intervention methods to help sedentary adults become and stay more physically active. It became apparent that a flexible, lifestyle approach to physical activity also is a valid way to help sedentary adults become more active and fit. The convergence of the new public health recommendations and new approaches to physical activity interventions has led to an increased interest in developing and evaluating alternative approaches of exercise programming.

The Physical Activity Intervention series is composed of texts, written by the leading researchers in the field, that provide specific and evidence-based methods for physical activity interventions. These books include practical suggestions, examples, forms, questionnaires, and specific intervention techniques that can be applied in field settings. Many health professionals who provide exercise advice and offer exercise programs use the traditional frequency, intensity, and time (FIT) approach to exercise prescription. Although this exercise prescription is valid, many people are reluctant to go to a fitness facility or participate in such programs. There is a need for alternative programs based on the new physical activity recommendation and the use of behavioral intervention techniques.

The books in this series provide information, techniques, and support to the many health professionals—clinical exercise physiologists, nutritionists, physicians, fitness center exercise leaders, public health workers, and health promotion experts—who are looking for alternative ways to promote physical activity that do not require a rigid application of the FIT approach. The Cooper Institute developed this Physical Activity Intervention series to meet this need.

The Physical Activity Intervention series includes books that focus on the implementation of theory-based physical activity interventions in the public health setting, after-school programs for children and youth, evaluation of physical activity interventions, the motivational readiness for change model, and focused interventions for other special populations such as older adults and those with chronic disease. Each book will be valuable in its own right, but as the series grows it will provide an integrated collection of materials that can be used for planning, developing, implementing, and evaluating physical activity interventions in a variety of settings for diverse populations.

I hope that the books in this series are useful to you. I will be delighted to receive your feedback, including recommendations for additional topics. Good luck in your crucial efforts to make our population more active, fit, and healthy.

Steven N. Blair
Series Editor
The Cooper Institute

The purpose of this book is to translate theories and concepts from behavioral science research into a handbook useful for health professionals who are involved in planning, developing, implementing, or evaluating physical activity programs. Our hope is that *Motivating People to Be Physically Active* will be useful for you if you are a personal trainer, an employee at a health club or community center, a staff member at a community or federal agency, or if any aspect of your job involves helping individuals to increase their motivation for behavior change, especially behavior change related to physical activity. We have tried to fill this book with practical tools, ideas, and methods that you can readily use no matter how much you do or do not know about the field of psychology and behavior change.

You may choose to read this book through in its entirety, or you may choose to read just the chapters that are most relevant for your work. However, we hope that you will become familiar with the concepts regarding motivational readiness presented in this book so that you can use it as a reference handbook for ideas and strategies to put those ideas into practice. The various skills, tools, and strategies presented here can be used in individual, group, workplace, or community settings.

While the aim of *Motivating People to Be Physically Active* is to provide you with knowledge, skills, and resources for working with healthy adults, you can apply the information presented here to whatever population segment you work with, including populations with chronic physical or psychological conditions.

In the first part of the book, we focus on the foundations of research on physical activity interventions, tools for measuring motivational readiness for behavior change, and mediators of behavior change. In chapter 1 we differentiate physical activity programs from other studies that pertain to exercise and fitness training. In chapter 2 we introduce the stages of motivational readiness for change model, the theoretical model that serves as the foundation of much of this book. In this chapter we also discuss how to measure motivational readiness for change. In chapter 3 we discuss other influential psychological theories and models and their application to physical activity interventions. In chapter 4 we describe mediators of change for physical activity behavior, which is what needs to change within a person before his or her physical activity behavior can change. In chapter 5 we describe how to measure these mediators of change. In chapter 6 we review physical activity intervention studies that have used the stages of motivational readiness model.

In part II we describe the assessment of patterns of physical activity and physical fitness, and we also look at applications of the stages of motivational readiness model to various settings. In chapter 7 we describe how to measure your clients' physical activity patterns and physical fitness. In chapters 8 through 11 we discuss how to apply the stages of motivational readiness model to individual, group, work-site, and community settings. We then discuss how you can apply these concepts to a specific population. Within these chapters we also provide some exercises and worksheets that you can use for your physical activity programs.

We wish you much success in your work helping people to be physically active. We applaud you for focusing your time and energy on this critically important area of health promotion and disease prevention.

ACKNOWLEDGMENTS

Before we mention the different people who have assisted us with this project, we first want to acknowledge that the writing of this book, while challenging, was fulfilling and sometimes downright fun because of the close professional and personal relationship we have. Working on this book while we each held down full-time jobs and parented young children was only possible because we supported and laughed with each other during the process.

There are several people who have assisted us with different aspects of this project. We thank Hazel Ouellette for helping to arrange time for us to communicate with each other, which is critical for a co-authored book! We thank Steven N. Blair, PED, for his helpful comments on an earlier version of the book. We thank Beth Lewis, PhD, Melissa Napolitano, PhD, Anna Albrecht, RN, MS, Andrea Dunn, PhD, and Jessica Whiteley, PhD, for their helpful comments on various sections of the book. We thank Laura Smith, MS, for her assistance in getting the paperwork for permissions completed. A special thanks to April Oberndorf for providing peace of mind. We would also like to thank Renee Thomas Pyrtel and Amanda Ewing at Human Kinetics for their editorial assistance throughout the writing of this book.

Photos

CREDITS

Theoretical Background and Tools for Measuring Motivational Readiness

PART

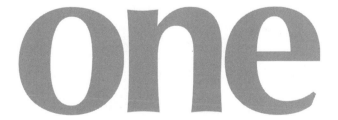

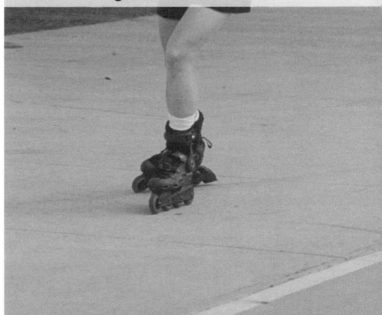

ONE

Description of Physical Activity Interventions

Sedentary living is a leading cause of poor quality of life, disability, and death in the United States and many other countries. Numerous well-conducted research studies on this topic have been completed over the past 50 years, providing convincing evidence of the important physiological and psychological changes that occur during and following exercise training programs. Data from these various studies have allowed researchers to develop guidelines for the amount of exercise needed to create and maintain these changes. Findings from these studies led the American College of Sports Medicine (ACSM) to develop the exercise prescription with which many of you are already quite familiar. That prescription was to exercise three to five times per week, training at 60 to 90 percent of maximum heart rate, for 20 to 60 minutes per session (ACSM, 1990). For many people, running is an activity that falls in this training range, while brisk walking does not.

Over the past decade numerous public health organizations—including the American Heart Association (AHA), the ACSM, the Centers for Disease Control and Prevention (CDC), the National Institutes of Health (NIH), and the Surgeon General—have released statements regarding the health benefits of an active lifestyle and the health consequences of a sedentary lifestyle (Fletcher et al., 1992; Pate et al., 1995; NIH, 1996; U.S. Department of Health and Human Services [USDHHS], 1996). The health benefits acquired through an active lifestyle are listed in figure 1.1. These statements are based on examinations of population-based studies that consistently found that physical activity or physical fitness reduces the risk of cardiovascular disease in a dose–response manner. That is, those who have the greatest fitness or participate in the greatest amount of physical activity have the lowest risk. These studies also found that those who perform moderate amounts of activity or who are moderately fit also have a large reduction in their risk for cardiovascular disease.

In addition to these population-based studies, several experimental studies led exercise scientists to examine the effect of intensity level as well as the minimum length of each bout of activity. A study by DeBusk and colleagues (1990) revealed that several short bouts (e.g., three 10-minute bouts) of moderate-intensity to vigorous-intensity activity in a day produced similar improvements in health-related outcomes to one longer bout (e.g., one 30-minute bout). Another study by Ebisu (1985) demonstrated that dividing exercise into three shorter sessions resulted in similar improvements in fitness and greater improvements in HDL

Reduced risk of heart disease, high blood pressure, and diabetes

Reduced risk of colon cancer

Healthy and strong bones

Less chance of catching colds and flu

Better weight management

Increased energy

Better sleep

Less anxiety and depression

Enhanced self-esteem

Figure 1.1 Benefits of physical activity.

cholesterol than one or two longer sessions. Thus, both vigorous- and moderate-intensity activity have important health implications, as do both continuous and accumulated bouts of activity.

These findings have resulted in health organizations' making recommendations for health-promoting physical activity: Adults should accumulate at least 30 minutes of at least moderate-intensity physical activity on most, preferably all, days of the week (Pate et al., 1995). Moderate-intensity activities are those that require exerting some effort but not pushing oneself as hard as more vigorous-intensity activities such as running. For example, we often tell clients that a good example of moderate-intensity activity is brisk walking, that is, walking with a purpose, as though you were late for a meeting, trying to catch a bus, or trying to get out of the cold. Figure 1.2 provides more examples of moderate-intensity physical activities.

Bicycling	Playing actively with children
Brisk walking (15–20 minutes per mile)	Playing volleyball
Dancing	Raking leaves
Gardening and yard work	Vacuuming a carpet
Golf (without a cart)	Washing and waxing a car
Hiking	

Figure 1.2 Examples of moderate-intensity physical activities.

Definitions of Physical Activity, Exercise, and Physical Fitness

Probably because many of us are used to the old recommendations, many health professionals and laypeople alike often use the terms *physical fitness, physical activity,* and *exercise* interchangeably, although their actual meanings are not the same. Perhaps you also substitute these terms for one another. However, notice that throughout this book we emphasize *physical activity* as opposed to exercise or physical fitness, in keeping with the new physical activity recommendations. We feel that the distinctions between these terms are critical, so let us clarify what each means before proceeding:

- *Physical fitness* is an outcome that can be attained through exercising at the frequency, intensity, and length of time prescribed by the ACSM (1995).

- The term *physical activity* refers to any bodily movement that results in the burning of calories (Caspersen, 1989).

- *Exercise* is actually a subcategory of physical activity; it is physical activity that is planned, structured, and repetitive.

The focus of this book is on developing programs that help individuals to increase *daily physical activity* rather than or in addition to planned exercise. This emphasis on physical activity as opposed to exercise recognizes that activities such as taking the stairs more often at work, raking leaves in the yard, or shooting baskets with the kids should be included as a successful outcome of programs such as those described in this book. A sedentary person who never liked vigorous "exercise" may be more accepting of a physical activity program that encourages strategies such as these.

Some strategies for meeting the CDC/ACSM public health recommendations include the following:

- Taking one 30-minute walk each day for at least five days of the week

- Taking one 30-minute walk on each weekend day and three 10-minute walks a day on at least three weekdays

- Doing three 10-minute bouts of activity on at least five days of the week (a sample day might include 10 minutes of digging in the garden, a 10-minute brisk walk to the post office, and 10 minutes of playing tag with the kids)

- Doing 30 minutes of heavy housework on one day, 30 minutes of heavy yard work on another day, and three days of accumulating at least 30 minutes of brisk walking in blocks of time that are at least 10 minutes in duration

You, as a health professional, are on the front line, working with people to change their behavior. Thus, these new recommendations are really written for you so that you can truly have a wide array of options for working with an individual, group, or community. We believe that most people will be much more responsive to your program offerings, individual coaching, or the like if you share with them this newer public health approach and the notion that they do not need to engage in intense, "no pain, no gain" workouts in order to reap all the benefits of a physically active lifestyle. In fact, by giving people the choice to accumulate their activity over the course of a day *or* to do it all at once, to do moderate-intensity activity such as brisk walking *or* more vigorous activities such as running, and to participate in physical activity at a gym, community center, *or* their own neighborhood, you give them enough tools to succeed at adopting and maintaining a physically active lifestyle, perhaps for the first time in their lives.

Physical Activity Interventions

The need for effective physical activity interventions is critical, given that 25 percent of the U.S. adult population, 40 to 50 million individuals, is sedentary and at high risk for chronic disease or functional limitations—a major public health problem (USDHHS, 1996). Moreover, since there are many social disparities (e.g., differing ages, income, and education levels) in the segments of the population who are sedentary, interventions that do not rely solely on costly face-to-face contact with a health or fitness professional are critical. Many people cannot afford to join a health club or community center. People in lower income brackets are also less likely to see a primary care doctor on a regular basis than those in higher income brackets. Thus, these individuals are not well served by current facilities and organizations. This has led behavioral scientists and public health researchers to develop effective interventions that can also be delivered through other channels, such as the Internet, telephone, pamphlets distributed within the community, and programs offered at the workplace (Marcus, Nigg, Riebe, & Forsyth, 2000).

Exercise training studies are typically conducted at a gym and supervised by health professionals. In exercise training studies, the goal is to determine the physiological effects of various amounts of exercise. Therefore, psychological theory is often not the framework on which these studies are based. In contrast, the goal for physical activity interventions is to help individuals change their behavior and replace sedentary pursuits with active ones. For example, helping people to learn to meet friends to go on walks or bike rides rather than for lunch or coffee might be one of the goals of a physical activity intervention. The goal of physical activity interventions is to work with individuals at reorienting their life to include physical activity.

Physical activity promoters are increasingly recognizing that to keep people active, they need to help them develop physical activity habits that fit their lifestyles. For example, for a person who works at the office from 8 A.M. until 8 P.M., having home exercise equipment may be the only way to structure the environment so that regular physical activity is an option. Of course, simply having exercise equipment in the environment does not provide the motivation for the individual to actually use it. For that, it may be important for the individual to learn to pair leisure activities he likes and perceives as important—such as watching the evening news, reading the newspaper, or listening to music—with use of the home exercise equipment. In this way, hopping onto the treadmill at 8:30 P.M. can be something to look forward to all day rather than one more thing to get through on a busy day.

Those who design physical activity interventions have also learned how important it is to help clients discover activities that they find enjoyable. Teaching people that activities they consider fun, such as dancing and gardening, can count toward the daily goal of accumulating 30 minutes of moderate-intensity activity is a great way to get people who otherwise might not take up regular exercise to at least consider doing so. Interventionists and program planners have also become aware of the need to design program offerings that are flexible enough to accommodate changes in their clients' life circumstances and routines. For example, jump-roping classes at health clubs and workplace wellness centers provide individuals the skill and the proper equipment to be physically active in any location.

Home-Based Versus Gym-Based Programs

It has become clear that giving individuals the choice of gym-based or home-based exercise programs has advantages. Home-based programs offer the opportunity for continuous or intermittent bouts of practical activities such as yard work, housework, and gardening. As a result of the difference in focus between home-based and gym-based programs, theoretical models that attempt to explain physical activity as a behavior and the factors that influence it have been central to physical activity intervention studies. For example, the stages of change approach, which examines an individual's motivation for changing her physical activity habits, the barriers that get in her way, the benefits she hopes to glean from an active lifestyle, and the specific strategies and techniques for becoming more active, may help her to achieve her goals. These parameters can be best addressed by applying psychological theories to the promotion of physically active lifestyles.

The Stages of Motivational Readiness for Change Model

The stages of motivational readiness for change model provides a framework for examining an individual's motivation for changing his physical activity habits, the barriers to change, the benefits of change, and specific strategies and techniques for promoting change.

The stages of motivational readiness for change model (Prochaska & DiClemente, 1983) is one of the four theoretical models highlighted in the recent Surgeon General's report on physical activity and health (USDHHS, 1996). This model has great utility for those who work with individuals, groups, and communities because it highlights the need to assess physical and psychological issues when designing programs and helps in the selection of strategies for behavior change that may be most useful for people with different levels of motivation to change. This theoretical framework is central to much of this book because it can help you understand how to motivate adults to be physically active.

References

American College of Sports Medicine. (1990). American College of Sports Medicine position stand: The recommended quantity and quality of exercise for developing and maintaining cardiorespiratory and muscular fitness in healthy adults. *Medicine and Science in Sports and Exercise, 22*(2), 265–274.

American College of Sports Medicine. (1995). *Guidelines for exercise testing and prescription* (5th ed.). Baltimore: Williams & Wilkins.

Caspersen, C.J. (1989). Physical activity epidemiology: Concepts, methods, and applications to exercise science. *Exercise and Sport Sciences Reviews, 17,* 423–473.

DeBusk, R.F., Stenestrand, U., Sheehan, M., & Haskell, W.L. (1990). Training effects of long versus short bouts of exercise in healthy subjects. *American Journal of Cardiology, 65,* 1010–1013.

Ebisu, T. (1985). Splitting the distance of endurance running on cardiovascular endurance and blood lipids. *Japanese Journal of Physical Education, 30,* 37–43.

Fletcher, G.F., Blair, S.N., Blumenthal, J., Caspersen, C., Chaitman, B., Epstein, S., et al. (1992). *American Heart Association position statement on exercise.* Dallas: American Heart Association.

Marcus, B.H., Nigg, C.R., Riebe, D., & Forsyth, L.H. (2000). Interactive communication strategies: Implications for population-based physical activity promotion. *American Journal of Preventive Medicine, 19*(2), 121–126.

NIH Consensus Development Panel on Physical Activity and Cardiovascular Health: NIH Consensus Conference. (1996). Physical activity and cardiovascular health. *Journal of the American Medical Association, 276,* 241–246.

Pate, R.R., Pratt, M., Blair, S.N., Haskell, W.L., Macera, C.A., Bouchard, C., et al. (1995). Physical activity and public health: A recommendation from the Centers for Disease Control and Prevention and the American College of Sports Medicine. *Journal of the American Medical Association, 273,* 402–407.

Prochaska, J.O., & DiClemente, C.C. (1983). The stages and processes of self-change in smoking: Towards an integrative model of change. *Journal of Consulting and Clinical Psychology, 51,* 390–395.

U.S. Department of Health and Human Services. (1996). *Physical activity and health: A report of the Surgeon General.* Atlanta, GA: Centers for Disease Control and Prevention, National Center for Chronic Disease Prevention and Health Promotion.

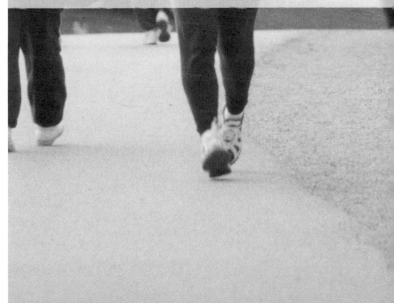

TWO

The Stages of Motivational Readiness for Change Model

As you may know, approximately 25 percent of the American population is sedentary. In addition, 60 percent of Americans report not participating in recommended amounts of physical activity (USDHHS, 1996). In the programs you manage, you may encounter people who participate in some activity, such as a Thursday night bowling or softball league or tennis with a friend on Saturdays, but do not participate in physical activity on a frequent enough basis to reap health benefits. Because so many people are either inactive or infrequently active, it is critical to find effective programs to help them start and stick with an active lifestyle.

Many of the techniques used to promote physical activity originated from psychological theories of motivation and behavior change. The stages of motivational readiness for change model, also known as the transtheoretical model or the stages of change model, evolved from the work of Dr. James Prochaska and Dr. Carlo DiClemente. Initially, they studied how people quit smoking on their own, without professional help (Prochaska & DiClemente, 1983). They were interested in learning how people change when they are not receiving help, thinking that this would provide valuable information to professionals who help others to change their health habits. Through their in-depth study of people who changed their smoking habits on their own, Drs. Prochaska and DiClemente learned that people moved through specific stages as they struggled to reduce the number of cigarettes they smoked or to quit smoking altogether. The model was initially labeled the transtheoretical model (Prochaska, 1979) because it was developed from many different psychological theories, such as social cognitive theory (Bandura, 1977) and learning theory (Skinner, 1953).

Motivational Readiness and the Stages of Change

The key concept in the model that Prochaska and DiClemente developed is that of *stages of change,* and thus many people refer to the model as the stages of change model. We call it the stages of motivational readiness for change model to emphasize that this model focuses on both motivation for change and actual behavior change. It acknowledges that when attempting to make long-lasting behavior changes, people vary in their levels of motivation to change, from no intention to change to actually making behavior changes.

This model posits that there are five stages of readiness for change. For physical activity, the stages are defined this way:

- Those in the *inactive and not thinking about becoming more active* stage (stage 1) include individuals who do no physical activity and do not intend to start in the next six months. This stage is hereafter referred to as *not thinking about change.*

- The *inactive and thinking about becoming more active* stage (stage 2) applies to people who do not participate in physical activity but intend to start in the next six months. This stage is hereafter referred to as *thinking about change.*

- Those in the *doing some physical activity* stage (stage 3) participate in some physical activity but not at levels meeting the CDC/ASCM (Pate et al., 1995) guidelines of accumulating at least 30 minutes of at least moderate-intensity physical activity on most, preferably all, days of the week (operationalized as at least five days a week) or the American College of Sports Medicine (1990) guidelines of at least 20 minutes of continuous vigorous exercise at least three days per week, and they may or may not intend to become more physically active.

- Individuals in the *doing enough physical activity* stage (stage 4) participate in recommended amounts of physical activity but have done so for less than six months and may or may not maintain this level of physical activity.

- Those in the *making physical activity a habit* stage (stage 5) have participated in recommended amounts of physical activity for six months or longer (Marcus & Simkin, 1993).

Movement through the stages is thought to be cyclical, rather than linear, as many individuals do not succeed in their efforts at starting and sticking with lifestyle changes (figure 2.1); in other words, people move back and forth through these different stages (Prochaska, DiClemente, & Norcross, 1992). For example, if an individual is in the thinking about change stage (stage 2) and moves straight into the doing enough physical activity stage (stage 4), accumulating at least 30 minutes of at least moderate-intensity activity at least five days a week, this may not result in long-lasting change. That is, if he skips over the stage of doing some physical activity (stage 3), he may not be adequately prepared for the rigors of daily activity, neither for the physical demand

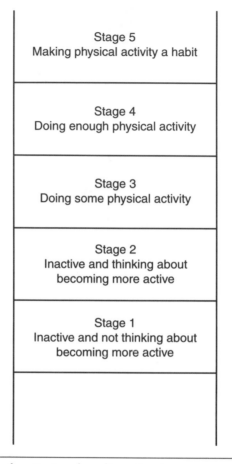

Figure 2.1 Stages of motivational readiness for change.

of that amount of activity nor for the time demand on his schedule. If he develops some foot or knee pain or decides that the two and a half hours per week he is devoting to walking takes too much time away from work, he may say, "The heck with this physical activity. It just doesn't fit into my life, so I am not going to do it." The risk is that not only will he slide back to an earlier stage, but in fact he may slide right back to the not thinking about change stage rather than the thinking about change stage.

This model is also referred to as cyclical because changing a habit often takes many cycles before success is attained. That is, an individual may need to make numerous attempts at behavior change before he is able to reach the making physical activity a habit stage (stage 5). You are probably quite familiar with the concept of one step forward and two steps back—this is often true for behavior change and may be quite frustrating for your clients.

Although the title of the fifth stage, making physical activity a habit, suggests that once a person reaches this level, she will maintain her physical activity for the long term, there is a strong likelihood that she may slide back to earlier stages for periods of time. This sliding back could be due to competing demands on her time, her health, or a myriad of other reasons. Fortunately, research has shown that once a person reaches this stage, she is more likely to slide back to doing some physical activity (stage 3) or at worst to thinking about change (stage 2) and not all the way back to not thinking about change (stage 1) (Marcus, Selby, Niaura, & Rossi, 1992).

It is not known whether a person needs to remain in making physical activity a habit (stage 5) for some critical period of time to reduce the risk of backsliding. In other words, it is not known whether there is a *termination* stage, that is when participating in physical activity on a regular basis is simply a permanent way of life, but it seems unlikely. Even if a person truly enjoys the activity in which he participates and has participated in it on a regular basis for many years, he still needs to remain vigilant to ensure that it happens on a regular basis. It never ceases to be an issue in his life. This is important for program planners and those working with clients to keep in mind as they help people to make short- and long-term goals for physical activity. The stages of change are summarized in table 2.1.

Table 2.1   The Stages of Motivational Readiness for Change

Stage number	Description
Stage 1	Inactive and not thinking about becoming more active
Stage 2	Inactive and thinking about becoming more active
Stage 3	Doing some physical activity
Stage 4	Doing enough physical activity*
Stage 5	Making physical activity a habit

*Accumulating at least 30 minutes of moderate-intensity physical activity at least five days per week.

Matching Treatment Strategies to Stages of Change

Most intervention programs are designed for individuals in the doing some physical activity stage (stage 3) or the doing enough physical activity stage (stage 4), that is, individuals who are already engaged in physical activity. However, more than half the population is not in either of these stages. Therefore, those of us interested in helping people to lead more active lives need to think about other types of programs to offer those in stage 1 and stage 2. They are the ones who are likely to most need to change, yet few opportunities for change are offered to them, and they are not motivated enough to seek out opportunities on their own.

We studied a sample of participants in a workplace health promotion project (Marcus, Rossi, Selby, Niaura, & Abrams, 1992), and classified 24 percent as in stage 1, 33 percent as in stage 2, 10 percent as in stage 3, 11 percent as in stage 4, and 22 percent as in stage 5. Other samples in the United States and Australia have shown similar percentages. Our studies and those of our colleagues in the United States, Australia, and Europe have demonstrated that when there is a mismatch between participants' stages of motivational readiness for change and the intervention strategy used, they are more likely to drop out of the program; even if they stay in, they are less likely to be successful at reaching their goals. For example, if a person still in stage 2 is given information appropriate for those in stage 4, such as specific tips on exercise programs, she may disregard the materials, intending to refer to them later, when or if she feels ready to start. This increases the chances that she will forget about the information she has received or decide that the program is not right for her because the material was not relevant to her level of motivation at that time. Matching treatment strategies to people's stage of motivational readiness for change improves the likelihood that they will regularly attend a program, increases their chances of meeting their short- and long-term goals, and decreases the likelihood that they will stop participating in the program or stop reading the materials provided.

Processes of Behavior Change

The stages of motivational readiness for change model also addresses the processes of behavior change (Prochaska, Velicer, DiClemente, & Fava, 1988). These processes of change are the strategies and techniques that individuals use to modify their behavior. The original work investigating the processes of change, like that investigating the stages of change, was conducted on smokers and has since been extended to physical activity.

The stages of change explain *when* people change, and the processes of change describe *how* people change. Determining which specific processes of change to focus on with a given client depends on that client's stage of motivational readiness for change. We developed a questionnaire about processes of change for physical activity (Marcus, Rossi, et al., 1992). Our research showed that for physical activity, all of the processes are important at all of the stages of change (Marcus, Rossi, et al., 1992). Nonetheless, it is not feasible to emphasize all processes at each contact with an individual, and thus key processes are usually selected based on a person's stage (Marcus, Bock, Pinto, Forsyth, Roberts, & Traficante, 1998).

Processes are divided into two categories: cognitive (involving thinking, attitudes, awareness) and behavioral (involving actions).

The cognitive processes of change regarding physical activity are

increasing knowledge,

being aware of risks,

caring about consequences to others,

comprehending benefits, and

increasing healthy opportunities.

The behavioral processes of change regarding physical activity are

substituting alternatives,

enlisting social support,

rewarding yourself,

committing yourself, and

reminding yourself.

The actual questions to assess these 10 processes of change (how much the client is using the process/strategy) are included in chapter 5. When people are in stage 2, they typically use mostly *cognitive* processes and some *behavioral* processes. Individuals in stage 4 typically use mostly *behavioral* processes and some *cognitive* processes. These strategies and techniques for helping people to change their behavior were

Table 2.2 The Processes of Change

Cognitive strategies	Behavioral strategies
Increasing knowledge Encourage your client to read and think think about physical activity.	**Substituting alternatives** Encourage your client to participate in physical activity when she is tired, stressed, or unlikely to want to be physically active.
Being aware of risks Provide your client with the message that being inactive is very unhealthy.	**Enlisting social support** Encourage your client to find a family member, friend, or co-worker who is willing and able to provide support for being active.
Caring about consequences to others Encourage your client to recognize how his inactivity affects his family, friends, and co-workers.	**Rewarding yourself** Encourage your client to praise himself and reward himself for being physically active.
Comprehending benefits Help your client to understand the personal benefits of being physically active.	**Committing yourself** Encourage your client to make promises, plans, and commitments to be active.
Increasing healthy opportunities Help your client to increase her awareness of opportunities to be physically active.	**Reminding yourself** Teach your client how to set up reminders to be active, such as keeping comfortable shoes in the car and at the office, ready to be used at any time.

derived from a variety of psychological theories and models and are often used in counseling (Prochaska, 1979). Table 2.2 illustrates how you can help clients to engage in the processes of change.

Programs based on the stages of motivational readiness for change model match treatment to the individual's stage of readiness for change. For example, a stage-matched physical activity promotion intervention for individuals in the early stages of change (stage 1 or stage 2) might focus on increasing use of the cognitive processes. Thus, the program might address topics such as increasing awareness of the benefits of physical activity and encouraging thinking about becoming active. Materials designed for individuals in the later stages (stages 3, 4, and 5) can focus more on the behavioral processes. Such materials might encourage individuals to begin exercising and suggest strategies for maintaining an active lifestyle, such as rewarding oneself for reaching an activity goal or putting reminders to be active around home and the workplace.

It is helpful to work with clients on increasing their self-confidence regarding their ability to become and stay physically active (Bandura, 1977). It is usually important to help clients understand more about the benefits of becoming physically active. Finally, since behavior change is not an easy process, it is also helpful to work with clients on understanding and overcoming their personal barriers to behavior change (Janis & Mann, 1977). Often components that address self-confidence, benefits, and barriers are used in combination with the stages and processes of change in an individual, group, workplace, or community program. More information about self-confidence, benefits, and barriers is provided in chapters 3 and 4. Information on measuring a client's stage of change is presented later in this chapter; information on measuring processes of change, self-confidence, barriers, and benefits is also provided in chapter 5.

Questionnaires

We now describe how to measure the stages of motivational readiness for change using a questionnaire. First, we describe the questionnaire, and then we discuss the scoring of the questionnaire. The flowchart in figure 2.2 is a helpful visual aid for explaining the staging concept to your clients. You can simply copy the questionnaires in this chapter for use with your clients.

Studies that have looked at the stages-of-change questionnaire have found that people tend to get similar scores over a two-week period of time (Marcus, Selby, et al., 1992). This gives us increased confidence that this questionnaire is measuring an individual's intentions and actual behavior in general, not just at the moment in time when they are filling out the questionnaire. We also have found that the questionnaire is related to measures of actual physical activity (Marcus & Simkin, 1993). This is important because it means that there is a direct relationship between a person's stage of motivational readiness for change and the number of minutes he is physically active each week. There is also a relationship between moving forward one or more stages of change and increases in physical fitness (Dunn, Marcus, Kampert, Garcia, Kohl, & Blair, 1997).

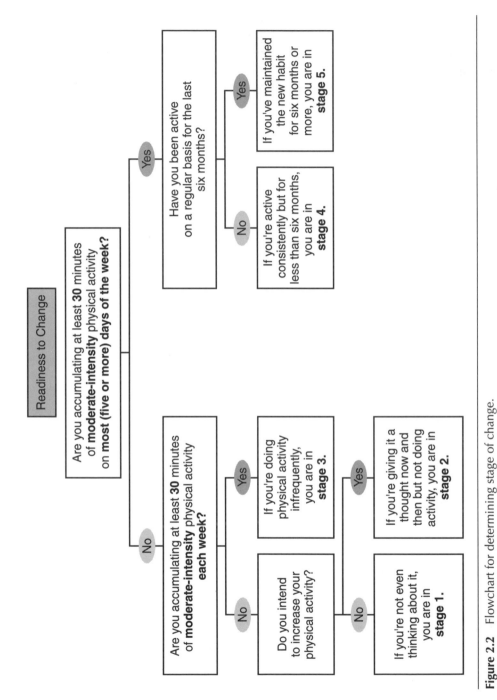

Figure 2.2 Flowchart for determining stage of change.

Reprinted, by permission, from S.N. Blair et al., 2001, *Active Living Every Day* (Champaign, IL: Human Kinetics), 9.

Physical Activity Stages of Change

For each of the following questions, please circle Yes or No. Please be sure to read the questions carefully.

Physical activity or exercise includes activities such as walking briskly, jogging, bicycling, swimming, or any other activity in which the exertion is at least as intense as these activities.

	No	Yes
1. I am currently physically active.	0	1
2. I intend to become more physically active in the next 6 months.	0	1

For activity to be *regular*, it must add up to a *total* of 30 minutes or more per day and be done at least 5 days per week. For example, you could take one 30-minute walk or take three 10-minute walks for a daily total of 30 minutes.

	No	Yes
3. I currently engage in *regular* physical activity.	0	1
4. I have been *regularly* physically active for the past 6 months.	0	1

Note: You may want to cover the following scoring algorithm before reproducing this questionnaire for a client.

Scoring Algorithm

If (question 1 = 0 and question 2 = 0), then you are at stage 1.

If (question 1 = 0 and question 2 = 1), then you are at stage 2.

If (question 1 = 1 and question 3 = 0), then you are at stage 3.

If (question 1 = 1, question 3 = 1, and question 4 = 0), then you are at stage 4.

If (question 1 = 1, question 3 = 1, and question 4 = 1), then you are at stage 5.

Marcus, Rossi, et al., 1992.

From *Motivating People to Be Physically Active,* by Bess H. Marcus and LeighAnn H. Forsyth, 2003, Human Kinetics, Champaign, IL.

Scoring the Stages-of-Change Questionnaire

For stages 1 and 2, clients should respond to questions 3 and 4 with zeros to ensure consistency in responses. In other words, clients who are inactive and either thinking about or not thinking about becoming active should give a "no" response to questions 3 and 4, because it is impossible to be not physically active and physically active at the same time. Occasionally, clients answer yes to both, which indicates that they have not read the questions carefully or that they do not understand them. In this case, you should clarify the meaning of these questions to your client.

The scoring algorithm determines clients' particular stage at the time they complete the questionnaire only. However, this questionnaire has been shown to be stable over a two-week period of time. When a client is found to be in stage 3 (doing some activity), 4 (doing enough activity), or 5 (making activity a habit), the second question (about whether he intends to increase his activity in the next six months) does not play a role in determining which stage he is in at the time the questionnaire is completed. This question is used to distinguish between clients in stage 1 (not thinking about becoming active) and stage 2 (thinking about becoming active). However, your client's intention to increase physical activity in the next six months can be highly relevant for intervention planning, and thus you may want to make a note of your client's intentions to increase activity. For example, if your client is in stage 3 (doing some activity) but answers that he is not planning to increase his activity over the next six months, you will probably want to ask him why he has sought your help. Perhaps he misunderstood the question. Or perhaps he only came to see you because his wife or his boss strongly encouraged him to do so, and he really has no intention of changing his behavior.

Other Variables

Following is a brief questionnaire that focuses on your client's current and past experiences with physical activity and the types of things that got in the way of your client's continuing with physical activity in the past. The information from this questionnaire can be useful as you plan an individual or group program for your client.

Physical Activity History

If you do *not* currently participate in physical activity, answer these questions:

1. How long has it been since you did *regular* physical activity or exercise?
    a. less than 6 months
    b. more than 6 months but less than 1 year
    c. more than 1 but less than 2 years
    d. more than 2 but less than 5 years
    e. more than 5 years but less than 10 years
    f. more than 10 years
    g. I have never been regularly physically active.

If you are *currently* physically active, answer the following questions:

1. How many days per week are you physically active? _____.

2. Approximately how many minutes are you physically active each time?
    _____.

3. How long have you been physically active at this level?_____.

4. What activities do you do? _____.

Answer the following questions whether or not you are currently physically active.

1. As an adult, were there ever times when you were physically active regularly for at least 3 months and then stopped being physically active for at least 3 months?

    a. yes   b. no

2. If yes, how many times? _____.

3. Regarding the most recent time, why did you stop your activity? (Please check as many as apply.)

Lack of time because of

___ work or school   ___ lack of physical activity partner
___ household duties   ___ lack of interest in physical activity
___ children   ___ health problems
___ social activities   ___ injury
___ spouse   ___ season or weather change
___ lack of money   ___ personal stress
___ lack of facilities   other: _____

From *Motivating People to Be Physically Active,* by Bess H. Marcus
and LeighAnn H. Forsyth, 2003, Human Kinetics, Champaign, IL.

References

American College of Sports Medicine. (1990). American College of Sports Medicine position stand: The recommended quantity and quality of exercise for developing and maintaining cardiorespiratory and muscular fitness in healthy adults. *Medicine and Science in Sports and Exercise, 22*(2), 265–274.

Bandura, A. (1977). Self-efficacy: Toward a unifying theory of behavior change. *Psychological Reviews, 84,* 192–215.

Dunn, A.L., Marcus, B.H., Kampert, J.B., Garcia, M.E., Kohl, H.W., III, & Blair, S.N. (1997). Reduction in cardiovascular disease risk factors: 6-month results from Project Active. *Preventive Medicine, 26,* 883–892.

Janis, I.L., & Mann, L. (1977). *Decision making: A psychological analysis of conflict, choice and commitment.* New York: Free Press.

Marcus, B.H., Bock, B.C., Pinto, B.M., Forsyth, L.H., Roberts, M.B., & Traficante, R.M. (1998). Efficacy of an individualized, motivationally-tailored physical activity intervention. *Annals of Behavioral Medicine, 20,* 174–180.

Marcus, B.H., Rossi, J.S., Selby, V.C., Niaura, R.S., & Abrams, D.B. (1992). The stages and processes of exercise adoption and maintenance in a worksite sample. *Health Psychology, 11,* 386–395.

Marcus, B.H., Selby, V.C., Niaura, R.S., & Rossi, J.S. (1992). Self-efficacy and the stages of exercise behavior change. *Research Quarterly for Exercise and Sport, 63,* 60–66.

Marcus, B.H., & Simkin, L.R. (1993). The stages of exercise behavior. *Journal of Sports Medicine and Physical Fitness, 33,* 83–88.

Pate, R.R., Pratt, M., Blair, S.N., Haskell, W.L., Macera, C.A., Bouchard, C., et al. (1995). Physical activity and public health: A recommendation from the Centers for Disease Control and Prevention and the American College of Sports Medicine. *Journal of the American Medical Association, 273,* 402–407.

Prochaska, J.O. (1979). *Systems of psychotherapy: A transtheoretical analysis.* Homewood, IL: Dorsey Press.

Prochaska, J.O., & DiClemente, C.C. (1983). The stages and processes of self-change in smoking: Towards an integrative model of change. *Journal of Consulting and Clinical Psychology, 51,* 390–395.

Prochaska, J.O., DiClemente, C.C., & Norcross, J.C. (1992). In search of how people change: Applications to addictive behaviors. *American Psychologist, 47,* 1102-1114.

Prochaska, J.O., Velicer, W.F., DiClemente, C.C., & Fava, J. (1988). Measuring processes of change: Applications to the cessation of smoking. *Journal of Consulting and Clinical Psychology, 56,* 520–528.

Skinner, B.F. (1953). *Science and human behavior.* New York: Free Press.

U.S. Department of Health and Human Services. (1996). *Physical activity and health: A report of the Surgeon General.* Atlanta, GA: Centers for Disease Control and Prevention, National Center for Chronic Disease Prevention and Health Promotion.

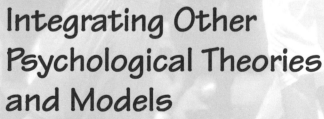

THREE

Integrating Other Psychological Theories and Models

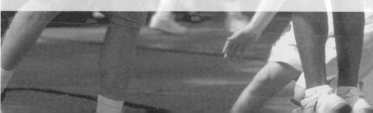

When you stop to think about it, physical activity is complex. It includes several types of behavior, such as walking, playing volleyball with the kids, or raking the leaves in the yard. It also includes more traditional types of exercise, such as jogging and aerobics. Several factors seem to influence whether a person is physically active, such as self-confidence, belief that one will gain something from their activity, support from family and friends, and enjoyment of active pursuits. Some health promoters have turned to psychological theories and models to better understand the many factors involved in starting to live an active lifestyle and maintaining physical activity behaviors. Theories from behavioral science also have been useful in developing, implementing, and evaluating various health promotion efforts. This chapter describes some psychological theories and models that can be useful when applied to physical activity and when developing strategies for helping clients to become more active. Several of the more promising theories are mentioned because no one model seems to fully explain physical activity and the ways in which we can most effectively help people to change this behavior. For example, it appears that some theories are more appropriate for looking at physical activity at the individual level, while others are applicable at the community level. A more comprehensive review of these theories and models can be found in chapter 6 of the 1996 Surgeon General's report *Physical Activity and Health* (USDHHS, 1996).

Learning Theory

Behavior modification and learning theories (Skinner, 1953) have been widely applied to physical activity behavior change. According to learning theory, a person is more likely to be physically active when the right circumstances are in place and pleasurable consequences occur as a result of physical activity (figure 3.1). For example, a client is more likely to be physically active when a place to exercise is readily available, he has time set aside, and he has already experienced a sense of accomplishment after squeezing in 30 minutes of activity on a previous day. In turn, if this client feels that activity is rewarding, he will be more likely to put in place the circumstances that will allow him to be active in the future.

Learning theory also acknowledges that when developing a new, complex behavior, such as becoming physically active, it is crucial to start with small steps and then progress slowly toward the desired result.

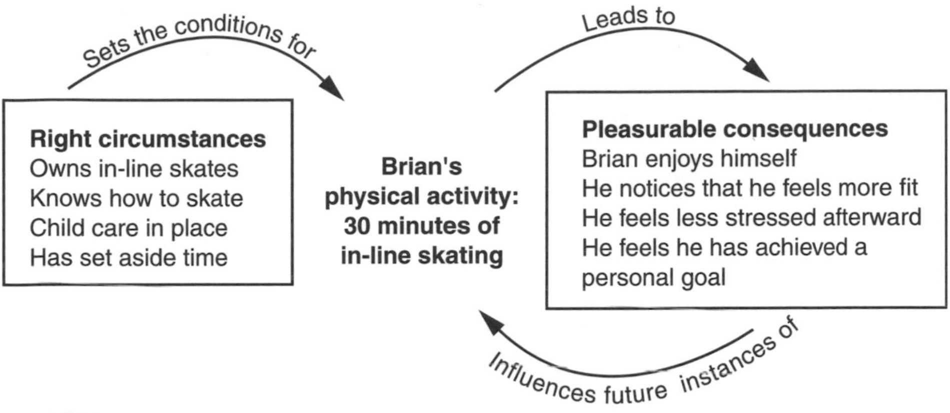

Figure 3.1 Learning theory.

This is called *shaping*. Often, newly physically active people start off by setting goals that are too difficult, such as walking every day for 45 minutes. Likewise, program developers often set up programs that are too frequent, long, or intense for those newly physically active such as three 60-minute kickboxing classes per week. As a result, the new exerciser becomes frustrated or injured and thus drops out before the physical activity habit is established. However, by setting smaller, achievable goals (e.g., starting off with a 10-minute walk once a week then gradually building to a 30-minute walk several times a week), the new exerciser can develop a sense of accomplishment and learn strategies for overcoming barriers that may have led to failure in the past. In other words, by starting off small, your client can develop a sense of mastery over several behaviors (scheduling time, taking a walk even when tired, asking a family member to look after the kids for half an hour) that are necessary for regular physical activity. As your client becomes skilled at each of these small steps, the goal is then gradually increased (e.g., adding five minutes of daily activity each week), and rewards are given for each step accomplished. However, it is critical that your client feel that it is okay, in fact preferable, to start off slowly. If she feels that this is a lesser approach to becoming more active and fit, she may disregard it, which will then undermine her relationship with you and increase the likelihood that she will set herself up for failure. For years people have been hearing "no pain, no gain," "go for the burn," and other messages that intense exercise in an all-or-none format is needed in order for benefits to be gleaned. We now know from the scientific literature that these extremes are not necessary for health. However, if your clients do not understand that your approach is consistent with the new recommendations and beneficial to their health, they may disregard your suggestions.

Learning theory also informs us that acquiring a new behavior typically requires frequent rewards and many pleasant consequences, at least in the beginning. This is particularly relevant to physical activity, which is often perceived as immediately punishing (e.g., time-consuming, painful, tiring), while many of its rewards (e.g., becoming healthier, feeling more energetic) do not occur for quite a while. Therefore, some programs have tried to increase immediate rewards by offering social praise and material rewards, such as cash for participation, until "natural" reinforcers such as stress relief, muscle tone, and so on are achieved. In fact, programs using reward strategies such as attendance lotteries, behavioral contracts, and tangible rewards (e.g., gift certificates for exercise clothes) have been found to increase regular exercise participation by as much as 75 percent (King et al., 1992). However, programs based on these types of extrinsic rewards do not seem to help people stay active over the long term (Glanz & Rimer, 1995). When a program that uses prizes to encourage participation or attendance ends, its participants tend to go back to their sedentary lifestyles. A more beneficial strategy might be a program allowing participants to earn points for every half hour of activity, which they can cash in for exercise clothes and gift certificates. This is a strategy that clients can implement on their own as a way to gain immediate reinforcement, and it can be continued over several months or even years. However, it is important to also incorporate strategies that enhance natural rewards from exercise (e.g., encouraging participants to set up their own support networks, helping participants find activities that they enjoy and can see themselves doing for a while) so that participants will be more likely to keep exercising after your formal involvement is over.

Although it is important for people to eventually experience intrinsic rewards (e.g., a feeling of accomplishment, other people's noticing weight loss, or increased vigor), this can take quite some time, especially for clients who do not tend to use intrinsic rewards in other aspects of their lives. Using reminders for physical activity also makes it more likely that a person will become physically active (figure 3.2). For example, Drs. Brownell, Stunkard, and Albaum (1980) found that simply posting a sign

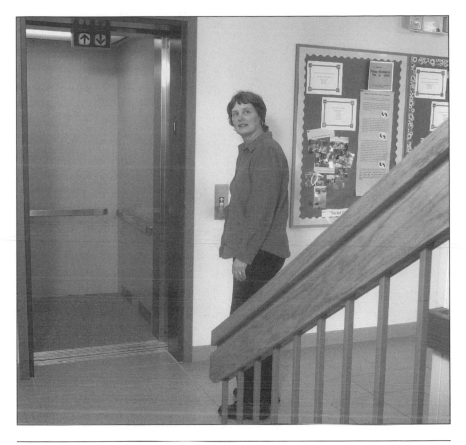

Figure 3.2 Taking the elevator is an unhealthy habit; taking the stairs is a healthy habit.

near the stairs and elevator with a cartoon of a healthy heart climbing the stairs encouraged people to use the stairs rather than the elevator.

Decision-Making Theory

Decision-making theory attempts to explain how people decide whether to engage in a particular behavior based on their comparison of the perceived benefits versus the perceived costs of the behavior (Janis & Mann, 1977). In other words, we are more likely to be active if we believe that the benefits of being active (e.g., improved health, stress relief) outweigh the costs (e.g., time taken away from other activities, getting hot

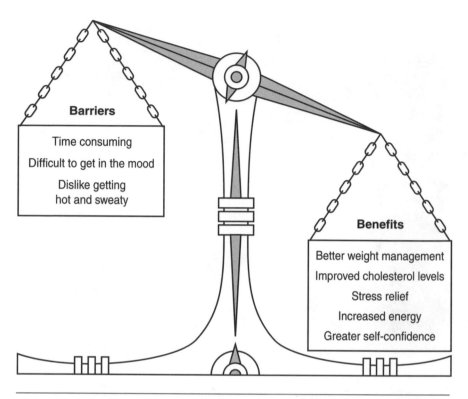

Figure 3.3 People are more likely to be motivated if they perceive the benefits to outweigh the barriers.

and sweaty) (figure 3.3). A person's weighing of the possible gains versus the difficulties or losses that will be experienced as a result of behavior change is often referred to as *decisional balance.*

People in the later stages of motivational readiness for change perceive more benefits of being physically active (more energy, less stress), while people in the earlier stages believe there are more disadvantages (uncomfortable, too time-consuming) than advantages (Marcus, Rakowski, & Rossi, 1992). One way you might use this theory in a program is to have your client write down what he thinks he will both gain and lose from participating in physical activity both in the short- and long-term. You can then use this list to begin discussing anticipated barriers and ways to increase perceived benefits (Marcus, Rakowski, et al., 1992; Wankel, 1984). Chapters 8 and 9 give other examples of how this theory can be used in designing individual and group programs.

Behavioral Choice Theory

Behavioral choice theory is based on decision-making theory but also incorporates research in the areas of learning, planning, and economics (Epstein, 1998). This theory tries to explain how individuals decide among the various behavioral options available to them and how they then use their time among various activities (both sedentary and active). According to this theory, people have a choice between being sedentary and physically active, and this choice is influenced by many factors, such as availability of physical activities versus sedentary behaviors, perceived benefits versus barriers, reinforcement (i.e., rewards, both tangible and perceived), and degree of effort (figure 3.4).

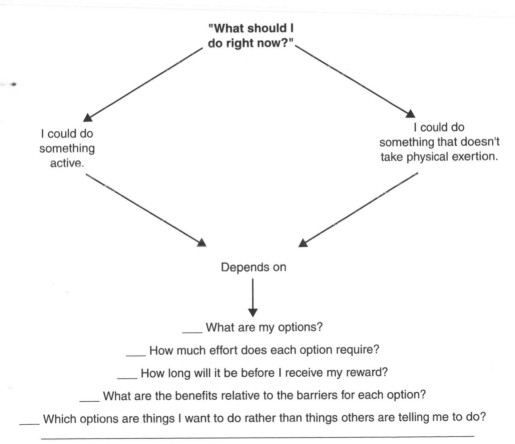

Figure 3.4 Behavioral choice theory.

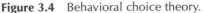

For example, reducing the accessibility of sedentary behaviors (e.g., parking spaces that are close to the building) and increasing the cost of being sedentary (e.g., a staircase close to the building's entrance but the elevator down the hall so that it actually takes more effort to find the elevator than simply taking the stairs) are both methods for reducing sedentary behaviors.

The choice to perform a behavior and enjoyment of a behavior depend partly on all the options that a client has available to him. For example, when your client comes home from a stressful day at work, he can plop down on the couch to watch TV, he can sit and talk to a friend on the phone, he can go out for a brisk walk, and so on. If you and he can come up with an option that is both enjoyable and readily available to him, you can influence him to choose an active pursuit rather than a sedentary one without having to throw the TV out or put a lock on the phone! For example, you might encourage your client to arrange to walk with a friend right after work as a way to relieve stress. You might encourage him to make his favorite sedentary activities dependent on doing some physical activity. For instance, if your client enjoys reading each night, you might encourage him to not do this sedentary behavior unless he has done 30 minutes of physical activity that day. Laboratory studies have shown that sedentary, obese children will spend time pedaling a stationary bike when pedaling the bike allows them access to their favorite sedentary behaviors such as playing video games or watching movies on the VCR (Saelens & Epstein, 1998). However, for this strategy to work, it is important that the sedentary behavior be one that the person enjoys or engages in often in everyday life (Saelens & Epstein, 1999).

Another important component of this theory is that for people to experience rewarding consequences as a result of physical activity, they need to feel that they freely chose to be active and are not active only to please someone else. If people perceive that they are being forced to initiate an activity program rather than choosing on their own to become more active, they may not be motivated to change their lifestyle to a more physically active one. Discussing how your client can personally benefit from physical activity or allowing him to set his own goals for physical activity rather than giving him the goal you think is best for him can help your client recognize that the choice of becoming active is his.

Finally, choosing an active over a sedentary behavior depends in part on the time delay between making the choice and reaping the benefits from that choice. For physical activity, many of the benefits (e.g., less risk of developing heart disease) are delayed, while the benefits of being sedentary (e.g., having fun watching a movie on television) are immediate. Therefore, it is important to encourage your client to look for immediate, but often overlooked, rewards of being active (e.g., feeling energized, the pleasure gained from doing something good for oneself, being a good role model to friends and family) and to keep in mind the long-term effects of sedentary behaviors that are often forgotten at the moment of choice.

Social Cognitive Theory

Social cognitive theory (Bandura, 1986) is one of the theories that has been applied most successfully to changing physical activity behavior. This theory proposes that behavior change is affected by interactions between the environment, personal factors, and attributes of the behavior itself (figure 3.5) (Bandura, 1986). In other words, each of these three forces may affect or be affected by the other two.

Furthermore, making physical activity a regular behavior can result from direct reinforcement. For example, you might praise a client who has stayed with her program for the last three months. Physical activity might also become habitual by observing the consequences of activity that others experience. For instance, Mary may decide to dust off her stationary bike after a friend describes how walking has helped her to feel less stressed and thereby to deal better with her kids, an issue which is also relevant for Mary.

A central concept in social cognitive theory is *self-efficacy*, or confidence in one's abilities to successfully perform a particular behavior. People's perceptions that they can perform successfully increases the likelihood that they will engage in that behavior. Self-efficacy is behavior specific; for example, a person may be confident that he can abstain from smoking but not feel that he will be able to stay physically active. To be even more specific, he may feel confident that he can maintain a walking program but not feel confident that he could get himself to a gym four times a week for a fitness class. Self-efficacy has been shown to be related to physical activity behavior (Sallis et al., 1989); therefore, it is important to evaluate and, if necessary, improve a client's self-efficacy for the type of activity you are targeting. Measuring self-efficacy is discussed in chapter 5; the questionnaire for self-efficacy can be adapted

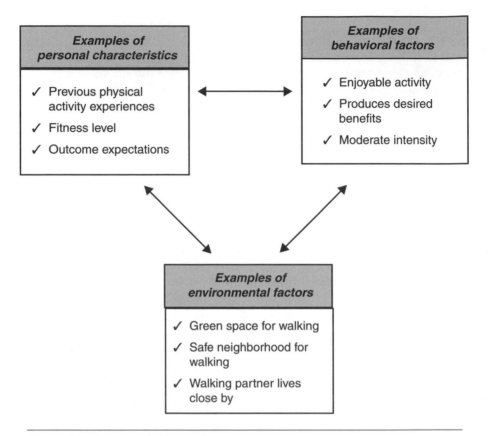

Figure 3.5   Reciprocal determinism.

for a specific type of physical activity behavior (e.g., walking). Strategies for enhancing self-efficacy are included throughout part II.

According to social cognitive theory, a person must also believe that positive outcomes *(outcome expectations)* will follow if she is physically active and that these positive outcomes (e.g., weight maintenance, lower cholesterol) outweigh any negative outcomes that might also be experienced (physical discomfort during activity). The person must value these positive outcomes, whether they be short term (e.g., feeling more energetic following physical activity) or long term (e.g., warding off heart disease or diabetes).

Ecological Model

The ecological model seeks to explain behavior and behavior change in relation to sociocultural and environmental variables. The basis of the ecological approach is that some environments restrict physical activities by promoting (and even demanding, in some cases) sedentary behaviors and limiting possible active pursuits (Sallis, Bauman, & Pratt, 1998). For example, many workplaces are designed in such a way as to limit opportunities for physical activity. Often the elevator is in a central location, while staircases are in the far corners of the building, and many workplaces do not contain exercise facilities or walking space nearby. Environments can be designed to foster activity by including more green spaces, bike paths, and staircases that are safe, attractive, and easily accessible. This model states that it is important to develop physical environments and policies that support activity, in addition to helping individuals develop personal skills, because there are multiple levels of influence on physical activity (McLeroy, Bibeau, Steckler, & Glanz, 1988). Table 3.1 illustrates the various levels of influence.

To successfully change physical activity behavior, the program must be implemented on multiple levels. Programs that influence multiple levels and multiple settings are more likely to lead to greater changes and longer-lasting maintenance of physical activity (Sallis, et al., 1998). Furthermore, it is important to customize the program to the setting at hand. For example, an outdoor walking program in an unsafe neighborhood or one with few sidewalks is not likely to be successful for many people.

Table 3.1 Components of the Ecological Model

Personal factors	Social factors	Institutional factors	Community factors	Public policy
Psychological	Friends	Companies	Organization of physical activity resources	Tax breaks for healthy behaviors
Biological	Family	Schools	Activity-related events in place	Laws protecting green space
Developmental	Co-workers	Health care facilities	Safe walking, biking trails	Better insurance rates for fit individuals

Relapse Prevention Model

Although the relapse prevention model (figure 3.6) was originally developed to better understand people's difficulty with addictive behaviors, such as quitting smoking or drinking (Marlatt & Gordon, 1985), it also has been useful in understanding and intervening to increase physical activity. The appeal of the relapse prevention model is that it is especially geared toward maintaining change over the long term. This is particularly important for a behavior such as physical activity because continuing to be active over time is necessary to maintain benefits. In fact, that is probably the biggest challenge in promoting physical activity—it does not do much good for people if they do not stick with it. Research has shown that men who were athletes in college but then stopped being active were no healthier than men who had never been active (Paffenbarger, Hyde, Wing, & Hsieh, 1986). Programs based on the relapse prevention model help newly physically active people anticipate

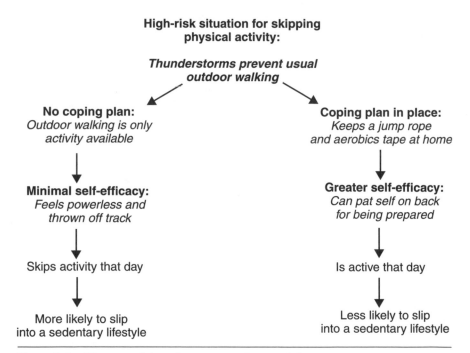

Figure 3.6 Diagram of the relapse prevention model.

Adapted, by permission, from G.A. Marlatt and J.R. Gordon, 1985, *Relapse prevention: Maintenance strategies in the treatment of addictive behaviors* (New York: Guilford Press), 38.

and plan for problems with sticking with their physical activity plans. Such problems might include depression and anxiety, injury, social pressure, difficulties with family members or friends, limited social support, low motivation, time pressure, and bad weather (USDHHS, 1996). This theory suggests that it is first important to identify situations that place a person at high risk for not being physically active (e.g., putting in a lot of hours at work) and then to develop a "game plan" to avoid or, if necessary, cope with each of these situations (e.g., take two or three 10-minute walks as work breaks). If a person finds herself in a situation in which she is at risk for not being active but uses her skills to overcome the temptation to be sedentary, her self-efficacy is likely to increase. On the other hand, if she fails to be active, she is probably going to feel less confident in her abilities to handle similar situations in the future.

Another helpful aspect of the relapse prevention model is that it encourages people to make a distinction between a *lapse* (e.g., a few days of not being physically active) and a *relapse* (an extended period of no physical activity) so that they do not fall prey to the *abstinence violation effect*. This term refers to people's tendency to give up altogether when they have "slipped." For example, a person who stops being active for a couple of weeks during a leisurely vacation may be disinclined to resume his activity program once he is home because he thinks to himself, "What's the use? I'm out of the routine." By acknowledging such a break in the physical activity habit as a normal but temporary occurrence, he will be more likely to tell himself, "Well, I had my break, but now it's time to start walking again." It is inevitable that your client will experience lapses, but these periods do not necessarily need to result in a return to a sedentary lifestyle. Your job may be to help your client plan for these potentially difficult situations.

CONCLUSION

You may have noticed that many of these ideas and program strategies are contained in the processes of change described in the previous chapter. For example, the behavioral processes of rewarding yourself and committing yourself come from learning theory, social cognitive theory, and the behavioral choice model. The cognitive process of comprehending the benefits comes from the behavioral choice model, decision-making theory, and social cognitive theory. Increasing healthy opportunities is directly related to the environmental approach derived from the ecological model. The relapse prevention model is related to the processes of reminding yourself and substituting alternatives.

Additionally, decisional balance, or the ratio of benefits to barriers of physical activity adoption (from decision-making theory) and self-efficacy (from social cognitive theory), have been shown to predict the stage of motivational readiness for physical activity (Marcus, Selby, Niaura, & Rossi, 1992; Marcus, Rakowski, et al., 1992) and physical activity behavior (Forsyth, Lewis, Pinto, Bock, Roberts, & Marcus, 2002; Sallis et al., 1989). These examples highlight the transtheoretical nature of the processes of change. We hope that, after reading this chapter, you also recognize that physical activity is not easily or completely described by any one theory or model. Table 3.2 illustrates how ideas from several theories can be translated into change strategies. In turn, these strategies can be combined to produce a more comprehensive program that is more likely to work. In other words, integrating the approaches suggested by multiple theories is more likely to lead to success than depending on any one model alone.

Table 3.2   Promising Psychological Models and Theories for Promoting Physical Activity

Theory or model	Relevant ideas	Program strategies
Learning theory	Shaping Reinforcement Stimulus control Extrinsic vs. intrinsic rewards	Self-monitoring Goal setting (both short- and long-term) Rewards Feedback
Decision-making theory	Perceived benefits Perceived barriers	Decisional balance sheet Removing barriers Problem solving Enhancing benefits
Behavioral choice theory	Reinforcement Benefits vs. barriers Perceived choice Availability of behavioral options	Rewards Decreasing sedentary options Including client in planning and decision making
Social cognitive theory	Self-efficacy Outcome expectations Direct reinforcement Observational learning	Skill building Setting achievable goals Identifying benefits Tangible rewards Social support

Theory or model	Relevant ideas	Program strategies
Ecological model	Personal skills Physical environment Policies	Self-management Matching program to environmental opportunities Altering physical environments to include more activity options
Relapse prevention model	High-risk situations Coping Abstinence violation effect	Planning Problem solving Identifying and changing negative thinking

Behavioral intervention research on physical activity is a new area of scientific investigation, with very few studies conducted before 1990. Nonetheless, we have learned a great deal about physical activity behavior and how to help sedentary individuals become and stay more active, and we can be confident that it is possible for physical activity programs to succeed. Part II describes ways to apply the program strategies suggested by the models and theories described in this chapter within a stages of change framework.

References

Bandura, A. (1986). *Social foundations of thought and action. A social cognitive theory.* Englewood Cliffs, NJ: Prentice Hall.

Brownell, K.D., Stunkard, A.J., & Albaum, J.M. (1980). Evaluation and modification of exercise patterns in the natural environment. *American Journal of Psychiatry, 137,* 1540–1545.

Epstein, L.H. (1998). Integrating theoretical approaches to promote physical activity. *American Journal of Preventive Medicine, 15,* 257–265.

Forsyth, L.H., Lewis, B., Pinto, B.M., Bock, B.C., Roberts, M., & Marcus B.H. (2002). *Social-cognitive mediators of physical activity behavior change in two print-based interventions.* Unpublished manuscript.

Glanz, K., & Rimer, B.K. (1995). *Theory at a glance: A guide for health promotion practice.* Bethesda, MD: U.S. Department of Health and Human Services, Public Health Service, National Institutes of Health, and National Cancer Institute.

Janis, I.L., & Mann, L. (1977). *Decision making: A psychological analysis of conflict, choice, and commitment.* New York: Collier Macmillan.

King, A.C., Blair, S.N., Bild, D.E., Dishman, R.K., Dubbert, P.M., Marcus, B.H., et al. (1992). Determinants of physical activity and interventions in adults. *Medicine and Science in Sports and Exercise, 24,* S221–S223.

Marcus, B.H., Rakowski, W., & Rossi, J.S. (1992). Assessing motivational readiness and decision-making for exercise. *Health Psychology, 11,* 257–261.

Marcus, B.H., Selby, V.C., Niaura, R.S., & Rossi, J.S. (1992). Self-efficacy and the stages of exercise behavior change. *Research Quarterly for Exercise and Sport, 63,* 60–66.

Marlatt, G.A., & Gordon, J.R. (1985). *Relapse prevention: Maintenance strategies in the treatment of addictive behaviors.* New York: Guilford Press.

McLeroy, K.R., Bibeau, D., Steckler, A., & Glanz, K. (1988). An ecological perspective on health promotion programs. *Health Education Quarterly, 15,* 351–377.

Paffenbarger, R.S., Hyde, R.T., Wing, A.L., & Hsieh, C. (1986). Physical activity, all-cause mortality, and longevity of college alumni. *New England Journal of Medicine, 314,* 605–613.

Sallis, J.F., Bauman, A., & Pratt, M. (1998). Environmental and policy interventions to promote physical activity. *American Journal of Preventive Medicine, 15,* 379–397.

Sallis, J.F., Hovell, L.M.R., Hofstetter, C.R., Faucher, P., Elder, J.P., Blanchard, J., et al. (1989). A multivariate study of determinants of vigorous exercise in a community sample. *Preventive Medicine, 18,* 20–34.

Saelens, B.E., & Epstein, L.H. (1998). Behavioral engineering of activity choice in obese children. *International Journal of Obesity, 22,* 275–277.

Saelens, B.E., & Epstein, L.H. (1999). The rate of sedentary activities determines the reinforcing value of physical activity. *Health Psychology, 18,* 655–659.

Skinner, B.F. (1953). *Science and human behavior.* New York: Free Press.

U.S. Department of Health and Human Services. (1996). *Physical activity and health: A report of the Surgeon General.* Atlanta, GA: Centers for Disease Control and Prevention, National Center for Chronic Disease Prevention and Health Promotion.

Wankel, L.M. (1984). Decision-making and social support strategies for increasing exercise involvement. *Journal of Cardiac Rehabilitation, 4,* 124–135.

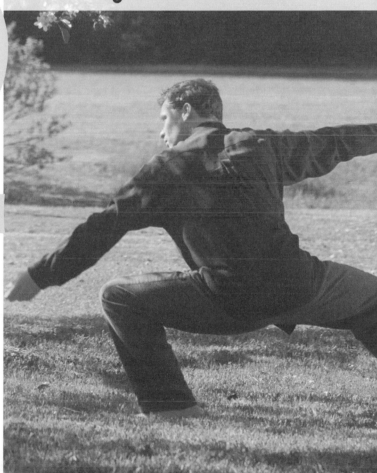

FOUR

Learning About Physical Activity Mediators

The previous chapter provided you with a description of some of the more promising psychological theories and models for physical activity programs. In this chapter we discuss specific factors derived from psychological theories and models that lead to, or *mediate,* behavior change. By paying attention to the mediators in your program, you can learn what strategies work best for changing physical activity and get ideas for improving future programs. First, we detail what a mediator is and why you might want to pay attention to the mediators in your program. Then we describe some of the mediators that have the most evidence for being important factors in changing physical activity behavior. We conclude the chapter by presenting some programs and the factors responsible for their success. This information should give you some ideas for designing and evaluating your own program.

Why Consider Mediators?

The psychological models and theories described in chapters 2 and 3 have generated ideas about what might encourage people to change their behavior. We call factors that lead to changes in behavior *mediators*. The theoretical model that serves as the basis for a program suggests which factors might serve as mediators. For example, a program based on social cognitive theory may focus on improving self-efficacy and outcome expectations for physical activity because changes in these factors are thought to lead to more physical activity, that is, they are thought to be mediators.

We are just beginning to discover the types of mediators that improve physical activity. Often when a program works, we really do not know what it was about the intervention that led to successful change (Baranowski, Anderson, & Carmack, 1998). However, it is worth considering what things may have produced (i.e., mediated) the change so that we can concentrate our efforts on the mediators that are likely to work best. For instance, if it appears that encouraging your client to reward herself more often after reaching her activity goals is partly responsible for your client's successfully becoming more active more days per week, that is helpful information to know when you design a program for someone else. It is our position that health promoters should consider not only measures of physical activity behavior or physical fitness when assessing the effectiveness of their interventions but also changes in relevant psychological and behavioral mediators of physical activity behavior change.

When people are already motivated to become more active (as are many volunteers who agree to participate in physical activity studies), many of our current interventions do appear to help people become more active than they would have if no intervention had been delivered at all (Baranowski et al., 1998). However, these improvements are not nearly as great as we would like—even for these motivated people! Studies of intervention effectiveness often report findings that are statistically significant, but the improvements in physical activity may not be enough to substantially improve health. As a health promoter, you know that the people we really need to help are the people who are *not* motivated to be active. For people in stage 1 (not thinking about change) or stage 2 (thinking about change), it is probably unrealistic for the intervention's goal to be to increase actual activity behavior to the public health criterion level or to enhance physical fitness. Instead, a more realistic goal for these clients would be to promote change in mediating factors that could, in turn, lead to more physical activity down the road. Depending on the person, "down the road" could be a few weeks, months, or years. Some may need a crystallizing moment, such as a birthday, anniversary, new job, or birth of a child; others will be able to set their own goals. Nonetheless, helping a less motivated person to even start thinking about how his health and outlook might improve if he were to be more active should be considered a successful outcome. Therefore, learning what needs to happen within that person for change to occur (i.e., discovering the mediators) is well worth your time and effort.

Moderators Versus Mediators

In research studies of physical activity mediators, the terms *mediator* and *moderator* are often used interchangeably (Baron & Kenny, 1986). Both are relevant and important, but their functions are quite different. The following two sections clarify these concepts and how they can be used.

Moderators

A moderator is a variable that can be used to divide participants into subgroups for whom the intervention works differently (Baron & Kenny, 1986). For example, Marcus, Bock, Pinto, Forsyth, Roberts, and Traficante

(1998) found that a motivationally tailored intervention was more effective for individuals in the earlier stages of motivational readiness (i.e., stage 1, not thinking about change, and stage 2, thinking about change) compared with a program that was not tailored to participants' motivational readiness for adopting physical activity. But both interventions were equally effective for individuals who were in stage 3 (doing some activity) (figure 4.1). In this case, stage of motivational readiness was a moderator of the tailored intervention's effectiveness. Age, sex, health status, and socioeconomic status are other variables that may be related to the effectiveness of a program and therefore may serve as moderators. For example, some interventions might work better for men than for women. In this case, sex serves as a moderator and should be considered when you recommend these interventions. Moderators tell us *who* will benefit most from a program, but they do not tell us *how* the intervention works. To determine this, we look at factors that change as a result of a program: the mediators.

Mediators

A mediator represents the mechanism through which the intervention is believed to influence physical activity behavior (figure 4.2). In con-

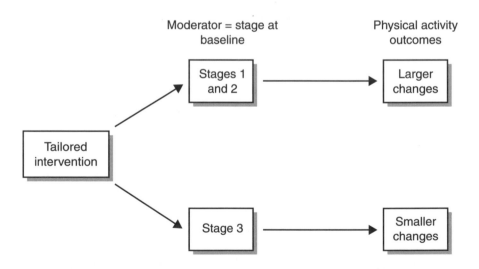

Figure 4.1 Example of baseline stage functioning as a moderator of intervention effectiveness.

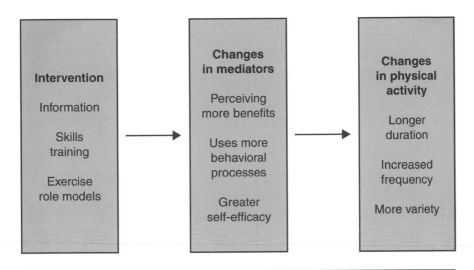

Figure 4.2   Examples of various mediators of physical activity behavior change.

trast to many moderators (e.g., age, sex), a mediator is always a factor that we can help a client change. Let us illustrate with an example. You might design a program based on the decision-making theory that attempts to help clients identify more benefits of becoming active and reduce the number of excuses they make for not being active. The theory is based on the assumption that if your clients associate more positives and fewer negatives with physical activity, they are more likely to become physically active. In this example, perceptions of positive and negative aspects of physical activity are believed to be mediators of behavior change. Prior to starting your program, you measure perceived benefits and perceived obstacles and find that your clients do indeed see more obstacles than benefits. After you complete your intervention and find that your clients have become much more active, you decide to again measure their perceived benefits and obstacles. If you find that your clients now see more benefits of being active and identify fewer excuses for staying sedentary, you have some evidence that your intervention's ability to improve decisional balance (i.e., ratio of perceived benefits to barriers; see chapter 3) helped your clients to become more active. At a higher level of sophistication, you might actually track changes in perceived benefits and perceived obstacles by repeated measurement of these variables to see whether changes occur first in these mediators or in physical activity behavior.

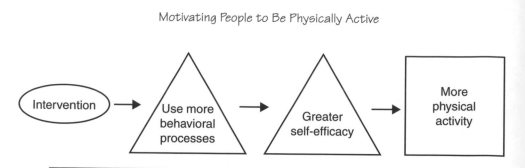

Figure 4.3 Physical activity mediators can also influence other mediators.

We are still in the early stages of identifying possible mediators of behavior change; the mediating process is a complicated one. When you hypothesize about possible mediators of your program's success, keep in mind that several mediators may be working at once (Baranowski et al., 1998). For example, self-efficacy, outcome expectations, and use of several behavior change processes may mediate the results of your intervention. Therefore, it is wise to consider and measure several possible mediators. To complicate things a bit further, mediating processes might work in a cascading sequence (Baranowski et al., 1998). For instance, an individual's ability to successfully use behavior change processes may help her feel more confident in her ability to be physically active (i.e., improve her self-efficacy), which may lead to her making more attempts to fit physical activity into her day (figure 4.3).

So far, we have found that changes in mediators never fully account for changes in physical activity behavior. There are many influences on physical activity level, such as genetics, environmental factors, and other forces that we have little or no control over (e.g., life events such as spraining an ankle), so it is impractical to think that we can completely predict physical activity outcomes through mediating variables. There are factors that influence physical activity that we have not discovered yet and others that we simply do not know how to measure. There are also factors that we may not have thought to measure and ones that we choose not to measure for one reason or another. As we mentioned in chapter 3, we have yet to find a theory that specifies every factor that may mediate changes in physical activity behavior. Thus, combining theories (the stages of motivational readiness model, social cognitive theory, decision-making theory, etc.) and building a program around several possible mediators (self-efficacy, perceived benefits, perceived barriers, processes of change, etc.) are likely to make the program more successful.

Mediators of Physical Activity

The remainder of this chapter focuses on mediators rather than moderators because these can be changed by an effective program. Following are descriptions of some of the constructs that have received empirical support as mediators of change for physical activity behavior. For information on specific instruments that have been developed to measure these constructs, please refer to chapter 5.

Self-Efficacy

Self-efficacy refers to confidence in one's ability to perform specific behaviors in specific situations (Bandura, 1986). For example, your client may have high self-efficacy (i.e., feel very confident) regarding his ability to maintain his walking program when he is in his usual environment. However, he may indicate lower self-efficacy for maintaining a walking program during a two-week vacation during which he plans to relax and take it easy. He may also remember that in the past during similar types of vacations he has let exercise go.

Another example illustrates how self-efficacy is also behavior specific. The same client may have a high level of self-efficacy for brisk walking because he enjoys this activity and, of course, knows how to do it. However, he may tell you that he feels less confident in his ability to maintain a regular swimming program because he has not done much swimming in the past and does not feel that he is good at it. Moreover, this activity requires changing clothing and traveling to a pool, which your client feels will be harder to do over the long term. In other words, people may vary in their self-efficacy for different types of physical activity, just as they are likely to vary in their self-efficacy for different health behaviors, such as eating healthy food or abstaining from smoking.

According to social cognitive theory, self-efficacy is the most important mediator of behavior change (Bandura, 1986). Many studies have found that self-efficacy is strongly related to physical activity behavior (Dishman & Sallis, 1994) and the best predictor of physical activity behavior (Sallis, Hovell, Hofstetter, & Barrington, 1992). In other words, improved self-efficacy leads to higher levels of physical activity at some later point in time (usually measured three to six months after the start of the program). Some studies have investigated self-efficacy

47

for physical activity across different situations, such as during vacation, when injured, during bad weather, and so on (Marcus, Selby, Niaura, & Rossi, 1992). Others have looked at self-efficacy for different components of being physically active, such as making time for activity and "sticking to it" (Sallis, Pinski, Grossman, Patterson, & Nader, 1988).

Social Support

Social support is believed to be another strong mediator of behavior change (Sarason & Sarason, 1985). There are different types of social support (Cohen, Mermelstein, Kamarck, & Hoberman, 1985). The first is *instrumental* support, which involves giving another person something tangible that will help in her efforts at behavior change. Examples of instrumental support include giving a person a ride to an exercise facility or giving your spouse a treadmill as a birthday gift. Another type of social support, *informational* support, involves helping a person make behavior changes by providing relevant information. For example, you might tell a friend about an upcoming fun run or talk to your sister about the processes you use to keep yourself motivated. *Emotional* support includes letting another person know that you care about him and how he is doing in his attempt to change his behavior. For example, when you call a friend or family member to see how he is faring with his attempt to be active for 20 minutes each day, you are offering emotional support. Finally, the fourth type of social support, *appraising,* involves providing feedback and encouragement to someone learning a new physical activity skill. For instance, an aerobics instructor provides this type of support when she tells a class participant that she has noticed the participant's improvement over the last few weeks. As these examples illustrate, social support can come from many sources, such as family members, friends, co-workers, exercise instructors, and other participants in an exercise class (USDHHS, 1996).

Decisional Balance

Decisional balance is the ratio of perceived benefits to barriers of change and comes from Janis and Mann's (1977) decision-making theory. With regard to physical activity behavior change, decisional balance refers to a person's perception of the benefits of physical activity compared to its negative aspects (Janis & Mann, 1977). Some people view physical activity in a positive light, while others focus more on its downside. Differences in decisional balance tend to correspond to different stages of motivational readiness. People in stage 1 (not thinking about change) perceive more barriers than benefits to change, while those in the later stages perceive more benefits than barriers (Marcus, Rakowski, & Rossi, 1992; Marcus & Owen, 1992). Some perceived barriers are environmental, such as bad weather, an unsafe neighborhood for walking, and a lack of available parks, sidewalks, and bicycle paths. Other barriers are more personal, such as feeling as though you do not have enough time or energy to be physically active after work. Fear of becoming injured, lack of motivation, and unhelpful friends or family members are other examples of personal barriers.

Behavior Change Processes

According to the stages of motivational readiness model, people use various cognitive and behavioral strategies and techniques to progress through the different stages of motivational readiness for change (DiClemente, Prochaska, Fairhurst, Velicer, Rossi, & Velasquez, 1991; Prochaska & DiClemente, 1983). Therefore, these processes are believed to be key mediators of behavior change. Examples of each of these processes of change are found in chapter 2. Studies have found that people in the later stages tend to use more of these processes than people in the earlier stages (Marcus, Rossi, Shelby, Niaura, & Abrams, 1992). Use of behavioral processes of change has been shown to significantly predict physical activity behavior (Calfas, Sallis, Oldenburg, & Ffrench, 1997; Dunn, Marcus, Kampert, Garcia, Kohl, & Blair, 1997; Forsyth, Lewis, Pinto, Bock, Roberts, & Marcus, 2002).

Outcome Expectations

This refers to the value a person places on the outcomes or consequences he believes will occur as a result of being physically active. Some of these outcomes occur immediately after being active, such as feeling energized. Other outcomes require being physically active for some time, such as losing weight or having more muscle tone. Specific outcome expectations that have been used to predict physical activity behavior include health benefits, improved body image, and psychological benefits such as stress reduction (Steinhardt & Dishman, 1989).

Enjoyment

It is not surprising that the people who say they enjoy physical activity tend to be the ones who become and stay active. While enjoyment of physical activity is not related to any specific theory, it consistently has been found to be associated with adult physical activity, stage of motivational readiness for change, and adherence to structured exercise programs (USDHHS, 1996). Therefore, it follows that if we can help a client enjoy physical activity more, that client is more likely to be active later on.

Empirical Support for Mediators

Although many physical activity programs are based on psychological theories and models, few studies test to see whether the program changed the theoretical constructs used to design the program (Baranowski et al., 1998). To do this, researchers first must determine whether the program changed possible mediators. For example, did a program based on social cognitive theory, which emphasizes self-efficacy, really help participants become more confident in their ability to become and stay active? The second step is then to determine whether changing the mediators led to participants' actually becoming more physically active. Some of the more recently published physical activity outcome trials have performed this type of analysis. Their results support the hypothesis that many of the possible mediators described in the preceding sections do help participants become more active.

Mediators in Physician-Based Programs

Project PACE (Provider-Based Assessment and Counseling for Exercise) was a well-conducted study that examined the effectiveness of brief counseling by primary-care providers for healthy adult outpatients (Calfas, Long, Sallis, Wooten, Pratt, & Patrick, 1996). The doctors' counseling was based on social cognitive theory and the stages of motivational readiness model and encouraged patients to use processes of change appropriate for their particular stage of motivational readiness for change. For example, if a brief assessment indicated that a patient was in stage 1 (not thinking about change) or stage 2 (thinking about change), then the physician might encourage that patient to read about the benefits of physical activity or to try one 10-minute walk that week. If the patient was in a later stage (e.g., stage 3, doing some physical activity), then the physician might counsel the patient to try increasing her activity to five or more 30-minute walks per week or to plan some type of reward for meeting her personal activity goal. Counseling was provided at well visits and followed up by a brief phone call for problem solving by a health educator two weeks afterward.

The activity levels of patients in practices that provided such counseling was compared with activity levels of patients in practices that did not offer any activity counseling. Patients who received counseling were found to have increased their physical activity significantly more than patients receiving standard care (Calfas et al., 1996). Examination of mediating variables found support for self-efficacy and use of behavioral processes of change as mediators of change for physical activity behavior, regardless of the program individuals received (Calfas et al., 1997).

Another physician-based program called Physically Active for Life (PAL) used the stages of motivational readiness model and social cognitive theory to design a program delivered to sedentary older adults (Pinto, Lynn, Marcus, DePue, & Goldstein, 2001). The PAL program also drew on information about the health behavior of middle-aged and older adults to help tailor the content of messages delivered by providers and printed materials for the patients. The program consisted of brief counseling delivered by physicians, physical activity prescriptions, and patient manuals based on the stages of motivational readiness model. Measures of physical activity conducted six weeks following the program showed that patients receiving the program were more physically active than patients receiving no program (Goldstein et al., 1999). However, these improvements did not last over time, as physical activity levels measured at eight months did not differ between groups. Similarly, changes in patients' decisional balance and patients' use of behavioral processes were found to produce improvements in motivational readiness at six weeks, but the effects were not maintained at 8 months (Pinto et al., 2001).

Mediators in Community-Based Programs

Project Active compared a counseling protocol regarding lifestyle activity with a traditional gym-based program for sedentary but healthy adults (Dunn et al., 1997; these programs are described in chapter 6). At the six-month assessment, 78 percent of participants in the lifestyle-activity group and 85 percent of participants in the structured-exercise group met the CDC/ACSM criteria for moderate-intensity activity (i.e., being physically active for at least 30 minutes on five or more days of the week). In both groups, greater use of cognitive and behavioral processes and improved self-efficacy led to these increases in physical activity. More specifically, substituting alternatives (e.g., doing something active such as playing ball with the children rather than sitting down in front of the TV with them), enlisting social support (e.g., talking to a friend or family member about exercise when you find yourself having trouble with it), rewarding oneself (e.g., consciously giving yourself a "pat on the back" or a small gift for going on a bike ride even though you did not feel like it), and committing oneself (e.g., telling yourself that you can keep active if you want to) served as mediators of behavior change. Identifying more benefits of activity than obstacles also led to higher activity rates for people in the lifestyle-activity group. In summary, the programs' ability to help participants (1) become more confident in their ability to be active, (2) use several behavioral processes of change, and (3) look for more positive aspects of exercise and focus less on the negative aspects helped participants to meet recommended levels of activity.

A study that looked at the effectiveness of two print-based programs delivered to a community sample of sedentary but healthy adults examined possible mediators of the programs' success (Forsyth et al., 2002). One program consisted of motivationally tailored manuals along with individualized feedback reports on participants' progress in self-reported activity, stage of motivational readiness, self-efficacy, decisional balance, and use of processes of change (Jump Start: A Community-Based Program is described in more detail in chapter 6). The feedback reports were about four pages long and provided each participant with information regarding any personal improvements or declines in these areas and his or her standing in comparison with others who had successfully become active.

The comparison program consisted of manuals from the American Heart Association (AHA) that were not tailored to participants in any way. These manuals were of similar length as the motivationally tailored manuals. The AHA manuals, while not personalized, provide excellent guidance on behavior change, advising starting gradually, setting goals, monitoring progress, and using other important behavioral processes for change. Materials were given at the start of the program and at one, three, and six months.

Both programs led to improvements in participants' physical activity levels. However, the group receiving the individually tailored feedback reported much more physical activity at six months than the comparison group (Marcus et al., 1998). Improved self-efficacy and using more behavioral processes of change led to more physical activity for both program groups (Forsyth et al., 2002). The behavioral processes—specifically, reminding oneself (e.g., laying out exercise clothes to remind you to exercise later), committing oneself, rewarding oneself, and substituting alternatives—seemed to help participants in the individually tailored feedback group become more active. Only two behavioral processes (committing oneself and substituting alternatives) were related to improved physical activity levels in the comparison group. The investigators hypothesized that this may have been the reason behind the individually tailored program's greater success in helping to improve activity levels (Forsyth et al., 2002). Therefore, providing people with individualized feedback about their ability to use behavioral processes may encourage them to use more of these processes than does giving the same message to all people. In turn, using more processes increases participants' chances of successfully becoming active at recommended levels. However, a good standard program does seem to help people make some behavior changes that lead to improved activity levels.

CONCLUSION

The findings across studies consistently suggest that programs that help people feel more confident in their ability to stay active and that encourage them to use more behavioral processes for change are more likely to improve actual physical activity behavior. Although cognitive processes of change (e.g., increasing knowledge, comprehending benefits) have not emerged as consistent mediators in the studies described in this chapter, this may be because these studies focused on predicting actual physical activity rather than intention to change, which characterizes the earlier stages of motivational readiness. However, working on intention to change may be critical for the clients who may be most neglected by the current program offerings in your setting. Furthermore, each of these studies focused on a limited number of potential mediating variables. For example, neither enjoyment nor outcome expectations were measured, but these factors may also have been partly responsible for physical activity improvements.

There are likely to be several other mediators that are yet untested but warrant further attention. For example, would a program that helps people make changes in their environment (e.g., moving the treadmill out of the spare bedroom and into main living areas or exercise space in the workplace) help them become more active? Does helping a client view her physical appearance (i.e., body image) more positively influence that client's activity levels down the road because she is less embarrassed to be seen exercising? Will including a client's family and friends in the program help that client to be more active? Considering factors like these, addressing them in your program, and then measuring them to see whether they change as a result of your program can help to open up the "black box" of changing physical activity behavior. The chapters in part II discuss strategies for influencing physical activity mediators.

References

Bandura, A. (1986). *Social foundations of thought and action: A social cognitive theory.* Englewood Cliffs, NJ: Prentice Hall.

Baranowski, T., Anderson, C., & Carmack, C. (1998). Mediating variable framework in physical activity interventions: How are we doing? How might we do better? *American Journal of Preventive Medicine, 14,* 266–297.

Baron, R.M., & Kenny, D.A. (1986). The moderator–mediator variable distinction in social psychological research: Conceptual, strategic, and statistical considerations. *Journal of Personality and Social Psychology, 51,* 1173–1182.

Calfas, K., Long, B.J., Sallis, J.F., Wooten, W.J., Pratt, M., & Patrick, K. (1996). A controlled trial of physician counseling to promote the adoption of physical activity. *Preventive Medicine, 25,* 225–233.

Calfas, K.J., Sallis, J.F., Oldenburg, B., & Ffrench, M. (1997). Mediators of change in physical activity following an intervention in primary care: PACE. *Preventive Medicine, 26,* 297–304.

Cohen, S., Mermelstein, R., Kamarck, T., & Hoberman, H.M. (1985). Measuring the functional components of social support. In I.G. Sarason & B.R. Sarason (Eds.), *Social support: Theory, research, and applications* (pp. 73–94). The Hague: Martinus Nijhoff.

DiClemente, C.C., Prochaska, J.O., Fairhurst, S.K., Velicer, W.F., Rossi, J.J., & Velasquez, M. (1991). The process of smoking cessation: An analysis of precontemplation, contemplation, and preparation stages of change. *Journal of Consulting and Clinical Psychology, 59,* 295–304.

Dishman, R.K., & Sallis, J.F. (1994). Determinants and interventions for physical activity and exercise. In C. Bouchard, R.J. Shephard, & T. Stephens (Eds.), *Physical activity, fitness, and health: International proceedings and consensus statement* (pp. 214–238). Champaign, IL: Human Kinetics.

Dunn, A.L., Marcus, B.H., Kampert, J.B., Garcia, M.E., Kohl, H.W., & Blair, S.N. (1997). Reduction in cardiovascular disease risk factors: 6-month results from Project Active. *Preventive Medicine, 26,* 883–892.

Forsyth, L.H., Lewis, B., Pinto, B.M., Bock, B.C., Roberts, M., & Marcus, B.H. (2002). *Social-cognitive mediators of physical activity behavior change in two print-based interventions.* Unpublished manuscript.

Goldstein, M.G., Pinto, B.M., Marcus, B.H., Lynn, H., Jette, A., Rakowski, W., et al. (1999). Physician-based physical activity counseling for middle-aged and older adults: A randomized trial. *Annals of Behavioral Medicine, 21,* 40–47.

Janis, I.L., & Mann, L. (1977). *Decision making: A psychological analysis of conflict, choice, and commitment.* New York: Collier Macmillan.

Marcus, B.H., Bock, B.C., Pinto, B.M., Forsyth, L.H., Roberts, M., & Traficante, R. (1998). Efficacy of individualized, motivationally tailored physical activity intervention. *Annals of Behavioral Medicine, 20,* 174–180.

Marcus, B.H., & Owen, N. (1992). Motivational readiness, self-efficacy and decision making for exercise. *Journal of Applied Social Psychology, 22* (1), 3–16.

Marcus, B.H., Rakowski, W., & Rossi, J.S. (1992). Assessing motivational readiness and decision-making for exercise. *Health Psychology, 11,* 257–261.

Marcus, B.H., Rossi, J.S., Shelby, V.C., Niaura, R.S., & Abrams, D.B. (1992). The stages and processes of exercise adoption and maintenance in a worksite sample. *Health Psychology, 11,* 386–395.

Marcus, B.H., Selby, V.C., Niaura, R.S., & Rossi, J.S. (1992). Self-efficacy and the stages of exercise behavior change. *Research Quarterly for Exercise and Sport, 63,* 60–66.

Pinto, B.M., Lynn, H., Marcus, B.H., DePue, J., & Goldstein, M.G. (2001). Physician-based activity counseling: Intervention effects on mediators of motivational readiness for exercise. *Annals of Behavioral Medicine, 23,* 2–10.

Prochaska, J.O., & DiClemente, C.C. (1983). Stages and processes of self-change of smoking: Towards an integrative model of change. *Journal of Consulting and Clinical Psychology, 51,* 390–395.

Sallis, J.F., Hovell, M.F., Hofstetter, C.R., & Barrington, E. (1992). Explanation of vigorous physical activity during two years using social learning variables. *Social Science and Medicine, 34,* 25–32.

Sallis, J.F., Pinski, R.B., Grossman, R.M., Patterson, T.L., & Nader, P.R. (1988). The development of self-efficacy scales for health-related diet and exercise behaviors. *Health Education Research, 3(3),* 283–292.

Sarason, I.G., & Sarason, B.R. (1985). *Social support: Theory, research, and applications.* The Hague: Martinus Nijhoff.

Steinhardt, M.A., & Dishman, R.K. (1989). Reliability and validity of expected outcomes and barriers for habitual physical activity. *Journal of Occupational Medicine, 31,* 536–546.

U.S. Department of Health and Human Services. (1996). *Physical activity and health: A report of the Surgeon General.* Atlanta, GA: Centers for Disease Control and Prevention, National Center for Chronic Disease Prevention and Health Promotion.

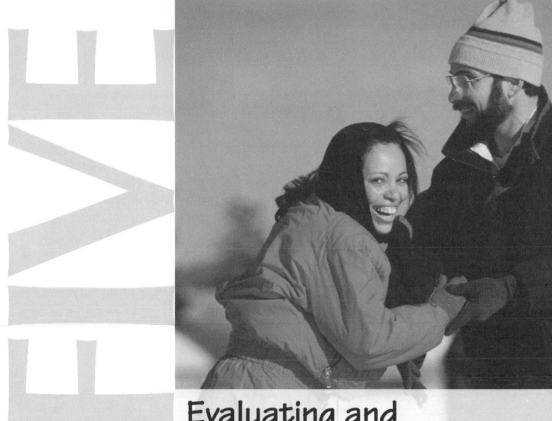

FIVE

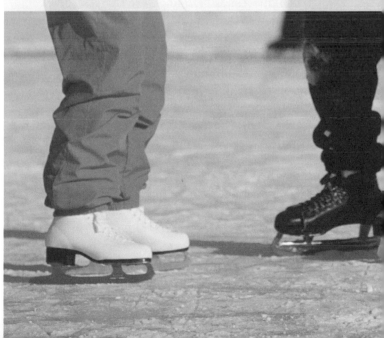

Evaluating and Measuring Physical Activity Mediators

In this chapter we describe how to measure the mediators of physical activity behavior that we discussed in chapter 4. We describe each questionnaire, provide you the actual questionnaire, and finally provide scoring instructions. You can simply photocopy the questionnaires for use with your clients. It is important to check that your client fills out these questionnaires completely and leaves no items unanswered.

We have chosen the questionnaires included in this chapter because they are based on key ideas from important theories and models of behavior change presented in chapters 2 through 4, specifically, processes of change, self-efficacy (confidence), decisional balance (decision making), social support, outcome expectations, and enjoyment. Additionally, these questionnaires have been shown to be useful for predicting behavior change in physical activity programs. We believe that these questionnaires can provide important information to share with your clients.

Processes of Change

A client's use of the processes of change for physical activity behavior can be measured with a questionnaire that we and our colleagues developed (Marcus, Rossi, Selby, Niaura, & Abrams, 1992). This questionnaire has been used in many exercise studies. When people's scores on these items increase, it is usually a good indicator that they are becoming more active (Dunn, Marcus, Kampert, Garcia, Kohl, & Blair, 1997). The processes of change are the strategies and techniques people use to change their thinking and their behavior; your clients are therefore likely to increase their use of many of the processes of change long before they are meeting national guidelines for a physically active lifestyle.

You may want to have clients complete this questionnaire every three months so that you can learn whether clients are making progress toward behavior change even if they are not meeting their specific physical activity goals. Recall that an individual's stage of motivation for change when he first comes to see you has a great impact on how quickly he increases his use of the different processes of change. The setting in which you work may also affect which processes of change increase first and how quickly they are put into use. For example, if you are a personal trainer at a health club, you are more likely to start working with clients on behavior change, and thus you are more likely to see increases in the behavioral processes of change. However, if you work at a community center, YMCA, or YWCA implementing a program like the Active Living Program (Blair, Dunn, Marcus, Carpenter, & Jaret, 2001), you may see changes in your clients' cognitive processes before change in their behavioral processes. Most published studies indicate that it is important for individuals to first increase their use of the cognitive processes and then of the behavioral processes. However, some studies indicate that the order is not important but rather that people need to increase their use of all (or most) of the processes of change in order to become and stay regularly active (refer to chapter 2 for examples of the processes of change) (Marcus, Rossi et al., 1992).

Processes of Change: Scoring
For each process, average the individual items by adding each group (shown in table 5.1) together and dividing by four. Do not score an individual process if fewer than three items were answered.

Table 5.1 Grouping Related Items on the Processes-of-Change Questionnaire

Process	Items
Increasing knowledge	5, 8, 17, 28
Being aware of risks	11, 12, 13, 14
Caring about consequences to others	30, 33, 34, 37
Comprehending benefits	15, 31, 35, 38
Increasing healthy opportunities	10, 22, 32, 36
Substituting alternatives	1, 21, 39, 40
Enlisting social support	16, 19, 24, 25
Rewarding oneself	7, 18, 20, 23
Committing oneself	2, 4, 6, 27
Reminding oneself	3, 9, 26, 29

For each process of change, the average score can range from 1 to 5. Table 5.2 shows typical average scores for the four items in each process group for people in each stage of motivational readiness for change. Please use this as a guide for understanding where your client is in the change process and on which areas to focus to help her successfully start and stick with a program of regular physical activity. If the survey

Table 5.2 Average Scores by Stage for the Processes-of-Change Questionnaire

Process	Stage				
	1	2	3	4	5
Increasing knowledge	1.88	2.57	2.76	3.11	2.99
Being aware of risks	1.92	2.41	2.26	2.72	2.46
Caring about consequences to others	1.82	2.43	2.46	2.74	2.47
Comprehending benefits	2.14	3.13	3.22	3.66	3.28
Increasing healthy opportunities	2.14	2.55	2.75	2.81	2.79
Substituting alternatives	1.71	2.24	2.72	3.35	3.55
Enlisting social support	1.78	2.25	2.42	2.80	2.64
Rewarding oneself	1.52	2.25	2.54	2.99	3.01
Committing oneself	2.08	2.94	3.17	3.83	3.68
Reminding oneself	1.42	1.85	2.02	2.30	2.20

results are similar on a number of processes, you can choose either a process or, in collaboration with your client, several processes to work on.

Processes of Change

Physical activity or exercise includes activities such as walking briskly, jogging, bicycling, swimming, or any other activity in which the exertion is at least as intense as these activities.

The following experiences can affect the exercise habits of some people. Think of any similar experiences you may currently have or have had during the **past month.** Then rate how frequently the event occurs. Please circle the number that best describes your answer for each experience.

How frequently does this occur?

> 1 = never
> 2 = seldom
> 3 = occasionally
> 4 = often
> 5 = repeatedly

1. Instead of remaining inactive I engage in some physical activity. 1 2 3 4 5

2. I tell myself I am able to be physically active if I want to. 1 2 3 4 5

3. I put things around my home to remind me to be physically active. 1 2 3 4 5

4. I tell myself that if I try hard enough I can be physically active. 1 2 3 4 5

5. I recall information people have personally given me on the benefits of physical activity. 1 2 3 4 5

6. I make commitments to be physically active. 1 2 3 4 5

7. I reward myself when I am physically active. 1 2 3 4 5

8. I think about information from articles and advertisements on how to make physical activity a regular part of my life. 1 2 3 4 5

9. I keep things around my place of work that remind me to be physically active. 1 2 3 4 5

(continued)

From *Motivating People to Be Physically Active,* by Bess H. Marcus and LeighAnn H. Forsyth, 2003, Human Kinetics, Champaign, IL.

10. I find society changing in ways that make it easier to be physically active.

1 2 3 4 5

11. Warnings about the health hazards of inactivity affect me emotionally.

1 2 3 4 5

12. Dramatic portrayals of the evils of inactivity affect me emotionally.

1 2 3 4 5

13. I react emotionally to warnings about an inactive lifestyle.

1 2 3 4 5

14. I worry that inactivity can be harmful to my body.

1 2 3 4 5

15. I am considering the idea that regular physical activity would make me a healthier, happier person to be around.

1 2 3 4 5

16. I have someone I can depend on when I am having problems with physcial activity.

1 2 3 4 5

17. I read articles about physical activity in an attempt to learn more about it.

1 2 3 4 5

18. I try to set realistic physical activity goals for myself rather than set myself up for failure by expecting too much.

1 2 3 4 5

19. I have a healthy friend who encourages me to be physically active when I don't feel up to it.

1 2 3 4 5

20. When I am physically active, I tell myself that I am being good to myself by taking care of my body.

1 2 3 4 5

21. The time I spend being physically active is my special time to relax and recover from the day's worries, not a task to get out of the way.

1 2 3 4 5

22. I am aware of more and more people encouraging me to be physically active these days.

1 2 3 4 5

23. I do something nice for myself for making efforts to be more physically active.

1 2 3 4 5

24. I have someone who points out my rationalizations for not being physically active.

1 2 3 4 5

From *Motivating People to Be Physically Active,* by Bess H. Marcus and LeighAnn H. Forsyth, 2003, Human Kinetics, Champaign, IL.

25. I have someone who provides feedback about my physical activity.   1 2 3 4 5

26. I remove things that contribute to my inactivity.   1 2 3 4 5

27. I am the only one responsible for my health, and only I can decide whether or not I will be physically active.   1 2 3 4 5

28. I look for information related to physical activity.   1 2 3 4 5

29. I avoid spending long periods of time in environments that promote inactivity.   1 2 3 4 5

30. I feel that I would be a better role model for others if I were regularly physically active.   1 2 3 4 5

31. I think about the type of person I will be if I am physically active.   1 2 3 4 5

32. I notice that more businesses are encouraging their employees to be physically active by offering fitness courses and time off to work out.   1 2 3 4 5

33. I wonder how my inactivity affects those people who are close to me.   1 2 3 4 5

34. I realize that I might be able to influence others to be healthier if I would be more physically active.   1 2 3 4 5

35. I get frustrated with myself when I am not physically active.   1 2 3 4 5

36. I am aware that many health clubs now provide babysitting services to their members.   1 2 3 4 5

37. Some of my close friends might be more physically active if I would.   1 2 3 4 5

38. I consider the fact that I would feel more confident in myself if I were regularly physically active.   1 2 3 4 5

39. When I feel tired I make myself be physically active anyway because I know I will feel better afterward.   1 2 3 4 5

40. When I'm feeling tense, I find physical activity a great way to relieve my worries.   1 2 3 4 5

Marcus, Rossi, et al. 1992.

From *Motivating People to Be Physically Active*, by Bess H. Marcus and LeighAnn H. Forsyth, 2003, Human Kinetics, Champaign, IL.

Self-Efficacy

We recommend measuring physical activity-specific self-efficacy with the questionnaire we and our colleagues developed (Marcus, Selby, Niaura, & Rossi, 1992). This brief, five-item self-efficacy questionnaire measures the major components of self-efficacy and has been used in many physical activity studies. People's self-efficacy scores almost always increase as they become more active. Again, we encourage you to administer this questionnaire to your clients every three months. If a client's score on this measure is not increasing, this is a red flag; you need to discuss this lack of self-efficacy with him because his belief that he cannot succeed with physical activity does not bode well for his becoming and staying active for life.

Self-Efficacy: Scoring

Calculate the score on the self-efficacy questionnaire by computing the average of all five items for each client. If any of the items are unanswered, have the client fill them in before scoring. A higher score on this measure indicates greater self-efficacy. Increased self-efficacy is important for an individual to adopt and maintain a program of regular physical activity.

Confidence (Self-Efficacy)

Physical activity or exercise includes activities such as walking briskly, jogging, bicycling, swimming, or any other activity in which the exertion is at least as intense as these activities.

Circle the number that indicates how confident you are that you could be physically active in each of the following situations:

Scale

      1 = not at all confident

      2 = slightly confident

      3 = moderately confident

      4 = very confident

      5 = extremely confident

1. When I am tired		1 2 3 4 5
2. When I am in a bad mood		1 2 3 4 5
3. When I feel I don't have time		1 2 3 4 5
4. When I am on vacation		1 2 3 4 5
5. When it is raining or snowing		1 2 3 4 5

Marcus, Selby, et al., 1992.

From *Motivating People to Be Physically Active,* by Bess H. Marcus and LeighAnn H. Forsyth, 2003, Human Kinetics, Champaign, IL.

Decisional Balance

We recommend measuring physical activity decision making with the decisional balance questionnaire that we and our colleagues developed (Marcus, Rakowski, & Rossi, 1992). This questionnaire measures a client's perceived benefits of and barriers to physical activity. Research has shown that for people to become more active, they need to see lots of benefits and not too many barriers to becoming more active. Over time, people tend to see more benefits than barriers to physical activity , and that is important to keeping them active over the long term.

Decisional Balance: Scoring
Compute the averages of the 10 pro items and of the 6 con items.

Pros = (item 1 + item 2 + item 4 + item 5 + item 6 + item 8 + item 9 + item 10 + item 12 + item 14)/10

Cons = (item 3 + item 7 + item 11 + item 13 + item 15 + item 16)/6

The difference in the averages (i.e., pros – cons) is the decisional balance score. Decisional balance scores greater than 0 show that your client sees more benefits than barriers to being active. The larger the score, the more benefits your client sees relative to barriers. A score less than 0 shows that your client sees more barriers than benefits of being physically active. The larger the negative score, the more barriers your client sees relative to benefits. As discussed in chapter 4, it is important to help your client see both more benefits and fewer barriers to physical activity. If your program is successful, you will likely see scores on this questionnaire move from negative to positive and then continue to rise.

Decisional Balance

Physical activity or exercise includes activities such as walking briskly, jogging, bicycling, swimming, or any other activity in which the exertion is at least as intense as these activities.

Please rate how important each of these statements is in your decision of whether to be physically active. In each case, think about how you feel **right now,** not how you have felt in the past or would like to feel.

Scale

　　1 = not at all important
　　2 = slightly important
　　3 = moderately important
　　4 = very important
　　5 = extremely important

1. I would have more energy for my family and friends if I were regularly physically active.　　1 2 3 4 5

2. Regular physical activity would help me relieve tension.　　1 2 3 4 5

3. I think I would be too tired to do my daily work after being physically active.　　1 2 3 4 5

4. I would feel more confident if I were regularly physically active.　　1 2 3 4 5

5. I would sleep more soundly if I were regularly physically active.　　1 2 3 4 5

6. I would feel good about myself if I kept my commitment to be regularly physically active.　　1 2 3 4 5

7. I would find it difficult to find a physical activity that I enjoy and that is not affected by bad weather.　　1 2 3 4 5

8. I would like my body better if I were regularly physically active.　　1 2 3 4 5

9. It would be easier for me to perform routine physical tasks if I were regularly physically active.　　1 2 3 4 5

(continued)

From *Motivating People to Be Physically Active,* by Bess H. Marcus and LeighAnn H. Forsyth, 2003, Human Kinetics, Champaign, IL.

10. I would feel less stressed if I were regularly physically active.   1 2 3 4 5

11. I feel uncomfortable when I am physically active because I get out of breath and my heart beats very fast.   1 2 3 4 5

12. I would feel more comfortable with my body if I were regularly physically active.   1 2 3 4 5

13. Regular physical activity would take too much of my time.   1 2 3 4 5

14. Regular physical activity would help me have a more positive outlook on life.   1 2 3 4 5

15. I would have less time for my family and friends if I were regularly physically active.   1 2 3 4 5

16. At the end of the day, I am too exhausted to be physically active.   1 2 3 4 5

Marcus, Rakowski, et al., 1992.

From *Motivating People to Be Physically Active,* by Bess H. Marcus and LeighAnn H. Forsyth, 2003, Human Kinetics, Champaign, IL.

Social Support

Physical activity research has looked at both general social support and social support specific to physical activity. A study comparing general social support and social support specific to physical activity found that they are quite distinct (Sallis, Grossman, Pinski, Patterson, & Nader, 1987). A person may feel that she has good social support for most areas of her life (e.g., a husband who helps with household responsibilities, friends and family members with whom she feels comfortable sharing her feelings and concerns) yet feel that there are few people who share her interest in physical activity, can give advice, or help with child care responsibilities so that she can make the time for physical activity. Therefore, we recommend using a questionnaire that was developed specifically to measure physical activity related social support from family and friends (Sallis et al., 1987). The client should answer each question for both family and friends. This instrument asks about exercise-related support obtained in the last three months, so you may want to administer it at three-month intervals to detect any changes. If your client receives a low score for social support from either friends or family, you may want to suggest some strategies for enhancing social support from these people because higher scores are associated with greater success in changing health habits and with better physical activity adherence (Sallis et al., 1987).

Social Support: Scoring
To score this measure, first invert the responses to questions 7 and 8 (1 = 5, 2 = 4, 3 = 3, 4 = 2, 5 = 1). Then sum all the items for family support and all the items for friend support separately. Higher scores reflect more perceived social support from these individuals.

Social Support for Physical Activity Scale

The following questions refer to social support for your physical activity.

The following is a list of things people might do or say to someone who is trying to do physical activity regularly. Please read and answer every question. If you are not physically active, then some of the questions may not apply to you.

Please rate each question *two times*. Under "Family," rate how often anyone living in your household has said or done what is described during the past three months. Under "Friends," rate how often your friends, acquaintances, or co-workers have said or done what is described during the past three months.

Please write *one* number from the following rating scale in each space:

    1 = none

    2 = rarely

    3 = a few times

    4 = often

    5 = very often

    0 = does not apply

	Family	Friends
1. Did physical activities with me.	____	____
2. Offered to do physical activities with me.	____	____
3. Gave me helpful reminders to be physically active (i.e., "Are you going to do your activity tonight?").	____	____
4. Gave me encouragement to stick with my activity program.	____	____
5. Changed their schedule so we could do physical activities together.	____	____
6. Discussed physical activity with me.	____	____
7. Complained about the time I spend doing physical activity.	____	____
8. Criticized me or made fun of me for doing physical activities.	____	____

From *Motivating People to Be Physically Active*, by Bess H. Marcus and LeighAnn H. Forsyth, 2003, Human Kinetics, Champaign, IL.

9. Gave me rewards for being physically active (i.e., gave me something I liked). _____ _____

10. Planned for physical activities on recreational outings. _____ _____

11. Helped plan events around my physical activities. _____ _____

12. Asked me for ideas on how they can be more physically active. _____ _____

13. Talked about how much they like to do physical activity. _____ _____

Reprinted, by permission, from J. Sallis et al., 1987, "The development of scales to measure social support for diet and exercise behaviors," *Preventive Medicine* 16:825-836.

From *Motivating People to Be Physically Active,* by Bess H. Marcus and LeighAnn H. Forsyth, 2003, Human Kinetics, Champaign, IL.

71

Outcome Expectations

As described in chapter 4, outcome expectations are beliefs that carrying out a specific behavior such as physical activity will lead to a desired outcome. Several research studies have found that people with greater outcome expectations for exercise are more likely to adopt and maintain regular physical activity. The brief Outcome Expectations for Exercise (OEE) scale (Resnick, Zimmerman, Orwig, Furstenberg, & Magaziner, 2000) can be used to measure your clients' expected benefits from activity. This scale asks about both the physical and mental benefits. If you find that your client has low expectations for physical activity, you should work with your client to identify some benefits he is likely to experience as a result of his activity. Doing so may help strengthen his outcome expectations, which in turn may improve his physical activity behavior.

Outcome Expectations: Scoring

This measure is scored by summing the ratings for all the items and dividing by 9 to get the average of all nine items. Scores can range from 1 to 5, with 1 indicating low outcome expectations for exercise and 5 suggesting high outcome expectations. Although the measure is used to obtain an overall score for outcome expectations, you can look at your client's scores on the individual items to determine the areas in which she feels she is less likely to benefit. Then you can focus on improving these areas.

Outcome Expectations for Exercise

The following are statements about the benefits of exercise (walking, jogging, swimming, biking, stretching, or lifting weights). State the degree to which you agree or disagree with these statements.

Exercise . . .	Strongly disagree	Disagree	Neither agree nor disagree	Agree	Strongly agree
1. Makes me feel better physically.	1	2	3	4	5
2. Makes my mood better in general.	1	2	3	4	5
3. Helps me feel less tired.	1	2	3	4	5
4. Makes my muscles stronger.	1	2	3	4	5
5. Is an activity I enjoy doing.	1	2	3	4	5
6. Gives me a sense of personal accomplishment.	1	2	3	4	5
7. Makes me more alert mentally.	1	2	3	4	5
8. Improves my endurance in performing my daily activities (such as personal care, cooking, shopping, light cleaning, taking out garbage).	1	2	3	4	5
9. Helps to strengthen my bones.	1	2	3	4	5

From *Motivating People to Be Physically Active*, by Bess H. Marcus and LeighAnn H. Forsyth, 2003, Human Kinetics, Champaign, IL.

Enjoyment

Many physical activity experts believe that feelings of enjoyment probably play an important role in helping people continue to be active over time (Dishman, Sallis, & Orenstein, 1985; Heinzelmann & Bagley, 1970; Martin & Dubbert, 1982; Wankel, 1985). Indeed, research has found that enjoyment is related to sticking with physical activity (Kendzierski & DeCarlo, 1991; King, Taylor, Haskell, & DeBusk, 1988). The Physical Activity Enjoyment Scale (PACES) is an 18-item measure that can be used to determine how enjoyable your client finds exercise. The developers of this measure say that it can be used for any given physical activity (Kendzierski & DeCarlo, 1991). You can help clients who score low on this measure to find activities that are more pleasurable, or you can adjust their activity so that it is less unpleasant (e.g., listening to music while being active, engaging in a moderate-intensity activity rather than a vigorous one, talking to a partner during activity).

Enjoyment: Scoring
For items 1, 4, 5, 7, 9, 10, 11, 13, 14, 16, and 17, assign point values as follows:

If client answered

1, give a score of 7

2, give a score of 6

3, give a score of 5

4, give a score of 4

5, give a score of 3

6, give a score of 2

7, give a score of 1

Then add all the items. Higher scores reflect greater enjoyment from physical activity. You can give this measure to your client periodically (e.g., every month or two) to see whether his enjoyment increases as he becomes more skilled and physically fit over time. Or you can have your client complete this questionnaire after you have made some suggestions for making physical activity more fun and your client has had a chance to try out your ideas. This can be a way of determining what makes activity more pleasurable for your client.

Physical Activity Enjoyment Scale

Please rate how you feel at the moment about physical activity. Below is a list of feelings with respect to physical activity. For each feeling, please mark the number that best describes you.

	1	2	3	4	5	6	7	
1. I enjoy it.	—	—	—	—	—	—	—	I hate it.
2. I feel bored.	—	—	—	—	—	—	—	I feel interested.
3. I dislike it.	—	—	—	—	—	—	—	I like it.
4. I find it pleasurable.	—	—	—	—	—	—	—	I find it unpleasurable.
5. I am very absorbed in physical activity.	—	—	—	—	—	—	—	I am not at all absorbed in physical activity.
6. It's no fun at all.	—	—	—	—	—	—	—	It's a lot of fun.
7. I find it energizing.	—	—	—	—	—	—	—	I find it tiring.
8. It makes me depressed.	—	—	—	—	—	—	—	It makes me happy.
9. It's very pleasant.	—	—	—	—	—	—	—	It's very unpleasant.
10. I feel good physically while doing it.	—	—	—	—	—	—	—	I feel bad physically while doing it.
11. It's very invigorating.	—	—	—	—	—	—	—	It's not at all invigorating.
12. I am very frustrated by it.	—	—	—	—	—	—	—	I am not at all frustrated by it.
13. It's very gratifying.	—	—	—	—	—	—	—	It's not at all gratifying.
14. It's very exhilarating.	—	—	—	—	—	—	—	It's not at all exhilarating.
15. It's not at all stimulating.	—	—	—	—	—	—	—	It's very stimulating.
16. It gives me a strong sense of accomplishment.	—	—	—	—	—	—	—	It does not give me any sense of accomplishment.
17. It's very refreshing.	—	—	—	—	—	—	—	It's not at all refreshing.
18. I feel as though I would rather be doing something else.	—	—	—	—	—	—	—	I feel as though there is nothing else I would rather be doing.

Adapted, by permission, from D. Kendzierski and K.J. DeCarlo, 1991, "Physical activity enjoyment scale: Two validation studies," *Journal of Sport & Exercise Psychology* 13(1):62-63.

From *Motivating People to Be Physically Active*, by Bess H. Marcus and LeighAnn H. Forsyth, 2003, Human Kinetics, Champaign, IL.

CONCLUSION

In this chapter we have given you tools to measure some important mediators of change in physical activity behavior. We provided the rationale for using the various questionnaires, the actual questionnaires, and instructions for scoring them. In the next chapter we put some of this information into use by telling you about some programs that have used the stages of motivational readiness for change approach to help individuals to become regularly active.

References

Blair, S.N., Dunn, A.L., Marcus, B.H., Carpenter, R.A., & Jaret, P. (2001). *Active living every day.* Champaign, IL: Human Kinetics.

Dishman, R.K., Sallis, J.F., & Orenstein, D.R. (1985). The determinants of physical activity and exercise. *Public Health Reports, 100,* 158–170.

Dunn, A.L., Marcus, B.H., Kampert, J.B., Garcia, M.E., Kohl, H.W., III, & Blair, S.N. (1997). Reduction in cardiovascular disease risk factors: 6-month results from Project Active. *Preventive Medicine, 26,* 883–892.

Heinzelmann, F., & Bagley, R.W. (1970). Response to physical activity programs and their effects on health behavior. *Public Health Reports, 85,* 905–911.

Kendzierski, D., & DeCarlo, K.J. (1991). Physical activity enjoyment scale: Two validation studies. *Journal of Sport and Exercise Psychology, 13,* 50–64.

King, A.C., Taylor, C.B., Haskell, W.L., & DeBusk, R.F. (1988). Strategies for increasing early adherence to and long-term maintenance of home-based exercise training in healthy middle-aged men and women. *American Journal of Cardiology, 61,* 628–632.

Marcus, B.H., Rakowski, W., & Rossi, J.S. (1992). Assessing motivational readiness and decision making for exercise. *Health Psychology, 11,* 257–261.

Marcus, B.H., Rossi, J.S., Selby, V.C., Niaura, R.S., & Abrams, D.B. (1992). The stages and processes of exercise adoption and maintenance in a worksite sample. *Health Psychology, 11,* 386–395.

Marcus, B.H., Selby, V.C., Niaura, R.S., & Rossi, J.S. (1992). Self-efficacy and the stages of exercise behavior change. *Research Quarterly for Exercise and Sport, 63,* 60–66.

Martin, J.E., & Dubbert, P.M. (1982). Exercise applications and promotion in behavioral medicine: Current status and future directions. *Journal of Consulting and Clinical Psychology, 50,* 1004–1017.

Resnick, B., Zimmerman, S.I., Orwig, D., Furstenberg, A., & Magaziner, J. (2000). Outcome expectations for exercise scale: Utility and psychometrics. *Journal of Gerontology: Social Sciences, 55B,* S352–S356.

Sallis, J.F, Grossman, R.M., Pinski, R.B., Patterson, T.L., & Nader, P.R. (1987). The development of scales to measure social support for diet and exercise behaviors. *Preventive Medicine, 16,* 825–836.

Wankel, L.M. (1985). Personal and situational factors affecting exercise involvement: The importance of enjoyment. *Research Quarterly for Exercise and Sport, 56,* 275–282.

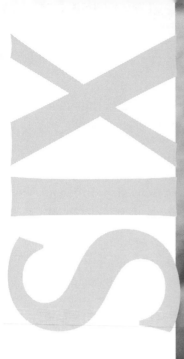

six

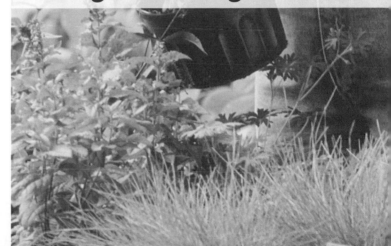

Successful Physical
Activity Interventions
Using the Stages Model

One concept that has been popular for years in the psychotherapy field is that of client–treatment matching. The idea that programs should be matched to the specific characteristics and needs of the client has also gained popularity in programs for quitting smoking and weight loss. However, we are just beginning to learn how to match physical activity programs to our target audience. This concept has been slow to reach the arena of exercise and physical activity programs, in part because leading a sedentary lifestyle has only recently begun to receive national recognition as a significant public health problem (USDHHS, 1996; Fletcher et al., 1992; Pate et al., 1995). There are a large number of gyms, community exercise programs, and health clubs in most urban and some rural communities, so resources are available for most people to exercise. Nevertheless, much of our population is sedentary, and most people who start an exercise program do not stick with it over the long term (Dishman, 1994). Therefore, the time seems right to consider client–program matching for the promotion of physical activity.

The stages of motivational readiness for change model is founded on the idea that people differ in their levels of readiness to change their behavior. Therefore, programs need to use differing strategies and techniques to bring about desired behavior changes. Additionally, program goals should differ based on the individual's or group's level of motivation for change. For example, the program goal for a client starting in stage 1 (not thinking about change) could be to help the client to begin to think about change by reading articles about the health, body image, and self-esteem benefits of physical activity and perhaps by taking a couple of 10-minute walks during the course of a week. In contrast, the goal of a program for a client in stage 3 (doing some physical activity) might include helping the client to take daily 10-minute walks and then building up to 30-minute walks on at least five days of the week.

In this chapter we describe a few different physical activity programs that have used the stages-of-change model. Earlier programs were able to attract people who were already physically active but had a harder time reaching those who were not. Part of the reason for this may have been the names used for previous programs. For example, one program offering was called "Get Fit." Not surprisingly, this program recruited people who were already active and wanted to become more fit or to maintain their fitness. Programs targeted at people in stage 2 have used different names, such as "Imagine Action," and "Jump Start to Health."

Imagine Action:
A Community-Based Program

The Imagine Action campaign was a community-wide physical activity program (Marcus, Banspach, Lefebvre, Rossi, Carleton, & Abrams, 1992). Participants were adults who enrolled through their workplaces or in response to advertisements. Potential participants received a description of the program with a letter explaining that if they were inactive or having difficulty staying active, this was a program designed for them. Respondents provided information about their activity level, name, address, sex, and birth date and were given a free T-shirt for enrolling. On average, participants were 42 years old, and 77 percent were women. At baseline, 39 percent were in stage 2 (thinking about change), 37 percent were in stage 3 (doing some physical activity), and 24 percent were in stage 4 (doing enough physical activity).

The program lasted six weeks and consisted of stage-matched self-help materials, a resource manual, and weekly fun walks and activity nights. The stage-matched materials were based on the exercise-adherence literature and informed by the stages of motivational readiness for change model, social cognitive theory, and decision-making theory. The manual for those in stage 2, called "What's in It for You," included information on increasing lifestyle physical activity (e.g., taking the stairs instead of the elevator, parking at the far end of the parking lot), considering the benefits (e.g., weight control) and barriers (e.g., activity takes too much time) of becoming more active, the social benefits of activity (e.g., meeting people in a class, walking with a friend), and rewarding oneself for increasing activity (e.g., buying a new CD as a reward for increasing from one to two walks per week).

The self-help manual for those in stage 3 was called "Ready for Action" because this group was participating in some activity but less than the goal of 30 minutes of moderate-intensity activity daily or 20 minutes of vigorous activity three to five times per week. This manual focused on the barriers and benefits of physical activity, setting short-term (e.g., making time for a daily walk) and longer-term activity goals (e.g., walking for 30 minutes five times per week), rewarding oneself for activity, time management to fit activity into a busy schedule (e.g., walking on treadmill while watching the news on television), and details on developing a walking program.

The self-help manual for those in stage 4 was called "Keep It Going" because these individuals had been regularly active only for a short time and thus were at risk for relapse to stage 3. This manual focused on troubleshooting situations that might lead to relapse (e.g., illness, injury, boredom), goal setting, rewarding oneself (both internal rewards such as self-praise and external rewards such as buying oneself flowers), cross-training to prevent boredom, avoiding injury, and gaining social support (e.g., finding people with whom to be active or who support an active lifestyle).

The resource manual described a wide variety of free and low-cost light-intensity, moderate-intensity, and vigorous physical activity options in the local community. The organized physical activity options included fun walks and appropriate free classes at local facilities, such as low-impact aerobics and volleyball for people who had never played.

Following the program, 30 percent of those in stage 2 and 61 percent of those in stage 3 at baseline progressed to stage 4 (doing enough physical activity), and an additional 31 percent who had been in stage 2 progressed to stage 3. Only 4 percent of those in stage 3 and 9 percent of those in stage 4 at the baseline slipped back to an earlier stage of motivational readiness. These findings demonstrate that a low-cost, relatively low-intensity program can produce important changes in physical activity.

Jump Start to Health: A Workplace-Based Study

The Jump Start to Health study examined the usefulness of a stage-matched physical activity program in the workplace for healthy, sedentary employees (Marcus, Emmons, et al., 1998). Employees were recruited through signs around the workplace about the study. Participating employees were placed at random in either a stage-matched self-help program or a non-stage-matched self-help program. The programs consisted of print materials delivered at the beginning of the study and one month later. Baseline stage of readiness and other information about physical activity habits was determined by having employees fill out a series of questionnaires in a private area at each participating workplace. At most of the workplaces, employees were given time off from work to fill out the questionnaires. At some workplaces, employees needed to use break time, lunchtime, or time after work. Free popcorn and beverages were available to employees who filled out questionnaires. Additionally, each employee who participated received a $1 Rhode Island State lottery ticket.

At the beginning of the study, individuals in the stage-matched group received manuals specifically tailored to their stage of motivational readiness for change (figure 6.1). One month later, these individuals received the manual matched to their current stage plus the manual for the next stage. The manual for those in stage 1 (not thinking about change) was titled "Do I Need This?" and focused on increasing awareness of the benefits of activity and the barriers that prevented participants from being active. Specific suggestions for starting an exercise routine were not provided in this manual. The manual for those thinking about change (stage 2), titled "Try It, You'll Like It," included a discussion of the reasons to stay inactive versus the reasons to become more active, learning to reward oneself, and setting realistic goals.

For those in stage 3 (doing some physical activity), "I'm on My Way" reviewed the benefits of activity, goal setting, tips on safe and enjoyable activities, and addressed obstacles to regular activity (e.g., lack of time, feeling too tired). "Keep It Going" provided information for those in stage 4 (doing enough physical activity) on topics such as the benefits of regular activity, staying motivated, rewarding oneself, enhancing confidence about being active, and overcoming obstacles. For those in stage 5 (making physical activity a habit), "I Won't Stop Now" emphasized the benefits of regular activity, avoiding injuries, goal setting, varying activities, rewarding oneself, and planning ahead. (These manuals can be ordered by calling 1-401-793-8176 or sending an e-mail to **LSExercise@lifespan.org**.)

Individuals in the non-stage-matched group received American Heart Association manuals (AHA, 1984a, 1984b, 1984c, 1984d, 1989). These print materials were selected as a comparison intervention because they are of excellent quality and readily available.

An examination of participants' responses to questionnaires at the beginning of the program and three months later revealed that more subjects in the stage-matched group than in the non-stage-matched group became more active (37 percent vs. 27 percent). The stage-matched approach was particularly effective for those who entered the program in stage 1, 2, or 3, which is noteworthy because these are the types of individuals who are most likely to be your clients.

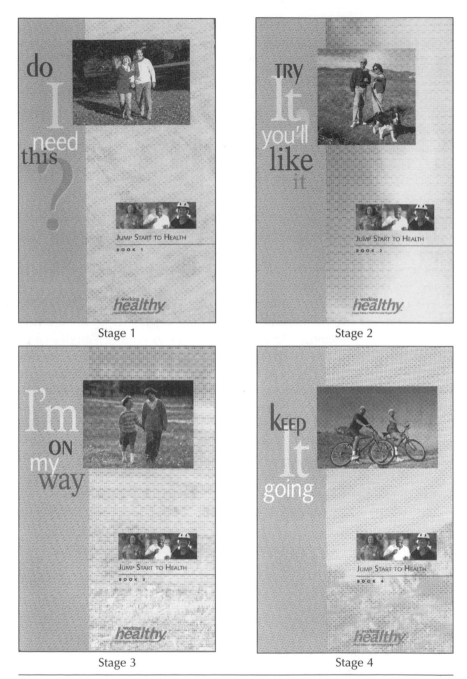

Stage 1

Stage 2

Stage 3

Stage 4

Figure 6.1 Manuals tailored to the different stages of motivational readiness for physical activity behavior change.

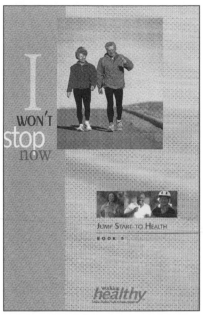
Stage 5

Figure 6.1 *(continued)*

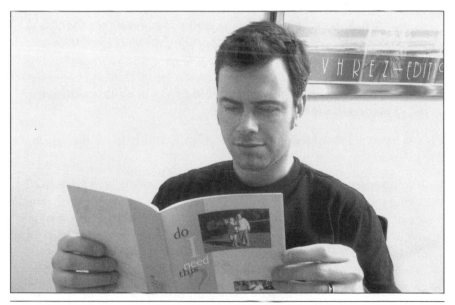
Participants in stage 1 may find this manual helpful.

Jump Start: A Community-Based Study

A community-based study compared a standard program (AHA 1984a, 1984b, 1984c, 1984d, 1989) to a stage-matched program that also provided individualized feedback to participants each time they filled out a questionnaire about their physical activity behavior (Marcus, Bock, Pinto, Forsyth, Roberts, & Traficante, 1998). The goal was to provide tailored comparisons between the behaviors of other successful individuals and of each participant. Additionally, feedback informed participants about how they had changed since the last time they filled out the questionnaires so that they understood whether they were moving forward, sliding backward, or doing about the same on a variety of strategies and techniques shown to be important for becoming a long-term physically active person.

Following are examples of two types of such feedback. The first example gives a comparison between the individual and other successful participants:

Your answers show that you are well aware of the benefits of regular exercise. This is something that you have in common with others in the program who have also made good progress. Since you already do some exercise, it's now important for you to gradually become more active and make exercise a more frequent and consistent part of your life. Now is the time to think about the things that could stop you from exercising regularly. Being prepared for the problems you may encounter is a big help in sticking to an exercise program. You will be better prepared to overcome obstacles by thinking about the kinds of thoughts and activities that will help you remain active during difficult periods.

This is an example of feedback regarding the individual's change since the prior assessment:

Your answers show that since we last heard from you, you have been taking more responsibility for your own health and well-being. You are also becoming more aware of the importance of believing in yourself and your ability to remain active. That's great! However, you are thinking a bit less about these issues than others who have succeeded in becoming and staying active.

To make more progress, try making a commitment to being more active. Think about the things you have done before, achievements you have made, goals you have reached. Try setting small goals for yourself, like going for a short walk or adding a few extra minutes of activity into each day—something you know you can do. This will help you strengthen your "can do" sense of accomplishment.

The individualized feedback concerned the topics of motivation, cognitive and behavioral strategies for becoming more active, barriers to and benefits from exercise, self-efficacy, and minutes of physical activity per week. Participants received printed reports and staged-matched manuals at the beginning of the program when they were first assessed by questionnaire and one, three, and six months later.

Results showed that those who received the individualized program were more likely to achieve recommended levels of physical activity (accumulating at least 30 minutes of physical activity per day at least five days per week) and were more likely to maintain that activity through a 12-month follow-up period than participants given standard materials promoting physical activity (Marcus, Bock, Pinto, Forsyth, Roberts, & Traficante, 1998; Bock, Marcus, Pinto, & Forsyth, 2001). Thus, this study shows that using materials matched to each individual's specific characteristics is helpful in increasing physical activity.

Project Active: A Community-Based Study

Project Active also was based on the stages of motivational readiness for change model; it had the benefit of following participants for 18 months after the initial phase of the program (Dunn, Marcus, Kampert, Garcia, Kohl, & Blair, 1999). Project Active was a two-year study that compared a lifestyle physical activity program (which encouraged participants to fit in 10-minute walks whenever they could) with a structured exercise program (which offered free membership at a beautiful gym). This study was conducted to compare the physical and psychological benefits of the lifestyle approach with those of a more traditional, structured exercise program in which it is more difficult to take into account an individual's motivation for change, unique barriers, and the like.

The lifestyle group members met for hour-long behaviorally oriented meetings each week that gradually decreased in frequency after the first four months of the program. Specific topics that were discussed are given in chapter 9; they included setting realistic goals for activity,

finding someone to support you so that you can be active, and

learning how to reward yourself for being active.

The structured-group participants were given a six-month membership to a fitness center and met with an exercise trainer who provided the type of support offered in many health clubs. These participants gradually increased their workouts to five days a week of at least 30 minutes of duration.

After the six-month program, both groups were much more active than at the beginning of the study (Dunn, Garcia, Marcus, Kampert, Kohl, & Blair, 1998). Additionally, 30% of participants were meeting the CDC/ACSM recommendations of participating in at least 30 minutes of moderate-intensity physical activity at least 5 days per week. After the entire two-year study period, both groups still showed improvements in energy expenditure and cardiorespiratory fitness compared with the beginning of the program (Dunn et al., 1999). Thus, in whatever setting you work, we encourage you to think broadly about the type of activity to encourage. The lifestyle approach may work best for many people, especially those starting out in stage 1 or 2. The curriculum used for Project Active is entitled *Active Living Every Day*, which is available through Human Kinetics.

CONCLUSION

Overall, the studies described in this chapter suggest that using a stage-matched approach helps people progress toward a more active lifestyle. These studies also demonstrate that matching an intervention to a participant's level of motivational readiness is a more effective approach than a simple one-treatment-fits-all approach in which all individuals receive the same information regardless of their motivation to change their activity levels. Personalizing information to the individual was found to be important. In the setting in which you work, accomplishing this personalization may be more or less feasible but nonetheless important.

Another important finding is that effective programs need not be the traditional gym-based ones with which you may be quite familiar. Lifestyle activity programs are also quite effective for the improvements in health and fitness that many of your clients are likely to want.

Here ends part I, in which we focused on the theoretical background and tools for measuring motivational readiness for change. In part II we focus on applying the stages of motivational readiness model in individual, group, work, and community settings.

References

American Heart Association. (1984a). *Dancing for a healthy heart.* Dallas: Author.

American Heart Association. (1984b). *Running for a healthy heart.* Dallas: Author.

American Heart Association. (1984c). *Swimming for a healthy heart.* Dallas: Author.

American Heart Association. (1984d). *Walking for a healthy heart.* Dallas: Author.

American Heart Association. (1989). *Cycling for a healthy heart.* Dallas: Author.

Bock, B.C., Marcus, B.H., Pinto, B., & Forsyth, L. (2001). Maintenance of physical activity following an individualized motivationally tailored intervention. *Annals of Behavioral Medicine, 23,* 79–87.

Dishman, R.K. (1994). *Advances in exercise adherence.* Champaign, IL: Human Kinetics.

Dunn, A.L., Garcia, M.E., Marcus, B.H., Kampert, J.B., Kohl, H.W., & Blair, S.N. (1998). Six-month physical activity and fitness changes in Project Active: A randomized trial. *Medicine and Science in Sports and Exercise, 30,* 1076–1083.

Dunn, A.L., Marcus, B.H., Kampert, J.B., Garcia, M.E., Kohl, H.W., III, & Blair, S. N. (1999). Comparison of lifestyle and structured interventions to increase physical activity and cardiorespiratory fitness: A randomized trial. *Journal of the American Medical Association, 281,* 327-334.

Fletcher, G.F., Blair, S.N., Blumenthal, J., Casperson, C., Chaitman, B., Epstein, S., et al. (1992). *American Heart Association position statement on exercise.* Dallas: American Heart Association.

Marcus, B.H., Banspach, S.W., Lefebvre, R.C., Rossi, J.S., Carleton, R.A., & Abrams, D.B. (1992). Using the stages of change model to increase the adoption of physical activity among community participants. *American Journal of Health Promotion, 6,* 424–429.

Marcus, B.H., Bock, B.C., Pinto, B.M., Forsyth, L.H., Roberts, M.B., & Traficante, R.M. (1998). Efficacy of an individualized, motivationally-tailored physical activity intervention. *Annals of Behavioral Medicine, 20,* 174–180.

Marcus, B.H., Emmons, K.M., Simkin-Silverman, L.R., Linnan, L.A., Taylor, E.R., Bock, B.C., et al. (1998). Evaluation of motivationally tailored vs. standard self-help physical activity interventions at the workplace. *American Journal of Health Promotion, 12,* 246–253.

Pate, R.R., Pratt, M., Blair, S.N., Haskell, W.L., Macera, C.A., Bouchard, C., et al. (1995). Physical activity and public health: A recommendation from the Centers for Disease Control and Prevention and the American College of Sports Medicine. *Journal of the American Medical Association, 273,* 402–407.

U.S. Department of Health and Human Services. (1996). *Physical activity and health: A report of the Surgeon General.* Atlanta, GA: Centers for Disease Control and Prevention, National Center for Chronic Disease Prevention and Health Promotion.

Applications

PART

two

SEVEN

Assessing Physical Activity Patterns and Physical Fitness

It is important for your clients to keep track of their participation in physical activity so that you know exactly what they are doing and can help them develop short- and long-term plans to reach their goals. Understanding patterns of behavior is an important first step. Once you understand how a client spends his time, you can begin to think of creative options to help him fit in some physical activity at times when he has been doing none and more activity at times when he has been doing a little. In this chapter we describe a variety of ways to track activity patterns. We discuss the use of the stages-of-change questionnaire, introduced in chapter 2, to examine patterns of physical activity behavior. We describe a system for tracking 10- and 30-minute bouts of light, moderate, or vigorous activity and another for recording everything done during the day and whether these activities are physically active or not. Next we introduce the idea of tracking physical activity habits with a pedometer. We describe using resting heart rate and time to walk half a mile (0.8 kilometers) to measure physical fitness. We conclude by mentioning strategies for using these tools with more than one person at a time. For more details about strategies for measuring physical activity, see the 1997 special issue of *Medicine and Science in Sports and Exercise* and the 2000 special issue of *Research Quarterly for Exercise and Sport,* which focus on this topic ("A Collection," 1997, "Measurement of PA," 2000).

In chapter 2 we discussed determining a client's stage of motivational readiness for change. Although the stages-of-change questionnaire does not allow you to learn about exact patterns of physical activity, such as times of day when a person was active or whether she performed her activity all at once or in multiple short bouts throughout the day, it does allow you to assess the person's current activity level and her intentions regarding future participation in physical activity. This questionnaire works well as a complement to other measures that provide detailed information about minutes of physical activity per day and types of activity performed. If you are working in a setting where global patterns of behavior and intention are most important, the stages-of-change questionnaire might be sufficient for your goals. This questionnaire is very brief, and studies have shown that scores on this measure correspond well with actual minutes of physical activity (Marcus & Simkin, 1993).

Tracking Physical Activity Behavior

Lack of time is a primary barrier for many people in their pursuit of a physically active lifestyle. This is why teaching your clients to keep track of how they spend their time is important. Once you understand how your client's time is spent, you can work with him to turn time spent in sedentary behavior and light activity into time spent in moderate-intensity physical activity. For example, you can suggest that your client replace time spent watching the kids play in the backyard with time spent bike riding or taking a nature walk with the kids. Thus you can help your client reorganize his time rather than take up more time for physical activity.

We know the health benefits associated only with moderate- and vigorous-intensity activity. We do not know about the health benefits associated with light activity. Table 7.1 shows some different categories of activities and examples of specific moderate-intensity and vigorous-intensity activities in each category.

You can have your client keep track of the amount of time she spends in these various categories of activities. It is best if she marks down her activity soon after performing the activity rather than trying to remember what she did for the whole week. Figure 7.4 on page 102 at the end of this chapter is a form your clients can use to keep track of this information. You can photocopy this form or use it as a starting point for creating your own with the information that you think is important for your client to record.

Table 7.1 Examples of Activities

Activity type	Moderate	Vigorous
Housework	Vacuuming carpet, cleaning windows, scrubbing floors	Moving furniture, shoveling snow, chopping wood
Occupation	Walking briskly at work	Using heavy tools, fire fighting, loading and unloading a truck, laying brick
Leisure	Ballroom dancing	Pop dancing
Gardening	Raking, mowing (push), weeding	Shoveling, carrying moderate to heavy loads, tilling, transplanting shrubs
Sports	Volleyball, table tennis, golf (without a cart), tai chi, Frisbee	Jumping rope, basketball, racquetball, soccer, mountain or rock climbing
Walking	Walking 15-20 minutes/mile	Running, stair climbing

Using the form in figure 7.4, a client can keep track of 10-minute bouts of activity, 30-minute bouts, or both, whichever you or he prefers. We recommend tracking 10-minute bouts of activity at a minimum because 10 minutes is a memorable amount of activity and thus the accuracy of recording should be fairly good. Your client can become more active over time by adding 10-minute bouts of activity each day until he accumulates 30 minutes each day. Your client instead may want to accumulate all 30 minutes in one bout of activity, which can also be reported on the form. Even though we don't know the benefits of light activity, you may want him also to record time spent in light activity because this information can give you some ideas on how to help him find time in the day to turn some of this light activity into moderate-intensity activity. For example, strolling in the mall window-shopping could be stepped up to walking at a moderate pace. If your client is not sure whether the activity was light, moderate, or vigorous, he should consider whether the effort was more like a slow walk at two miles (3.2 kilometers) per hour (light activity), a brisk walk at three to four miles (4.8–6.4 kilometers) per hour (moderate activity), or a run (vigorous activity).

At the end of each week, you or your client can add up the number of minutes checked for each activity category. You and your client can use this information to set realistic goals for improving your client's level of physical activity, to design a specific activity program, and to measure success at meeting goals.

In the example in figure 7.1, you can see that this person does a lot of light activity during the week but very little moderate or vigorous activity. Thus, one important strategy for working with this person is to examine which of the light activities could be performed at a moderate intensity. This client does not appear to have a time barrier; she is already spending time in activities. You could focus on helping her turn some of her light-intensity walking and gardening into moderate-intensity activity.

Time Tracking

To help your client find more time to be physically active, it is important to find out how he spends his work and leisure time. This information can help him find times in the day when he is sedentary and could do some physical activity. Further, it can aid him in finding bouts of activity that can be lengthened, for example, 2-minute bouts of activity

Activity	Intensity level	10-minute bouts	30-minute bouts	Total minutes
Housework	Light	*****		50
	Moderate/vigorous			0
Occupation	Light	*******	****	190
	Moderate/vigorous			0
Leisure	Light	****		40
	Moderate/vigorous			0
Gardening	Light	**		20
	Moderate/vigorous			0
Sports	Light			0
	Moderate/vigorous			0
Walking	Light	*********	*	120
	Moderate/vigorous	**		20
Stairs	Light	****		40
	Moderate/vigorous			0

Figure 7.1   Filled-out activity-tracking sheet.

Reprinted, by permission, from S.N. Blair et al., 2001, *Active Living Every Day* (Champaign, IL: Human Kinetics), 12.

that could be turned into 5-minute bouts and 5-minute bouts that could be turned into 10-minute bouts. Only by understanding his activity patterns can you help him to change these patterns. Have your client choose two weekdays and one weekend day in an upcoming week during which he will track his activities. Instruct him to carry a worksheet such as the one in figure 7.5 (on page 103 at the end of this chapter) on each of these three days and to record exactly what he does with his time. Figure 7.2 is a partially filled-out example.

After your client has recorded his activities, you can determine how many minutes he spends doing any type of physical activity and how many minutes he spends in sedentary pursuits (such as watching

Date: _____ **Day of week:** _____

Time slot	Activities, chores, errands, work, child care, leisure	Physically active? Yes	No
9:00 A.M. to 11:00 A.M.	Work at desk		25 minutes
	Attend meeting		30 minutes
	Walk to friend's desk and back	3 minutes	
	Walk to buy coffee and back	8 minutes	
	Walk to meeting	4 minutes	
	Work at desk		50 minutes
	Total time	**15 minutes**	**105 minutes**
11:00 A.M. to 1:00 P.M.	Walk to local deli and back with friend	10 minutes	
	Eat lunch with friend		20 minutes
	Walk back to desk	5 minutes	
	Work at desk		62 minutes
	Walk to buy coffee and back	8 minutes	
	Coffee break		10 minutes
	Return to office	5 minutes	
	Total time	**28 minutes**	**92 minutes**

Figure 7.2 Time-tracking example.

Reprinted, by permission, from S.N. Blair et al., 2001, *Active Living Every Day* (Champaign, IL: Human Kinetics), 48.

television or driving). The more specific your client can be, the more useful this activity will be for you both.

After your client tracks his physical activity habits, it is time to put this information to work to assist your client in becoming more active. First, look for patterns in the tracking forms that your client has filled out. Does your client tend to be sedentary for the entire workday? If so, suggesting a 10-minute walk once each workday might be a great way to help him on his way to a more active lifestyle. Another pattern to look for is time spent in light activity. Help your client to turn strolls into brisk walks, elevator rides into stair climbing, and light yard work into more vigorous yard work. The tracking forms are tools to help you individualize a program for your client—a program in which you know he can succeed!

Using a Step Counter

Step counters can be an excellent way to quantify amounts of activity. Many pedometers come with extra features such as calculators of distance covered or calories burned. These extra components are unnecessary and often inaccurate. The goal is for your client to increase her activity. If she gets too hung up on how far she has walked or how many calories she has burned, it may distract her from the goal and thus make meeting it less likely. Also, since distance and calorie calculations are often based on an average person, the values are often inaccurate for the individual using them. For example, if your client is short and has a small stride, the readings may be off. Your client is best served with a simple version that just counts steps. (The brand of step counter we prefer and use in our programs is Digi-Walker [**www.digiwalker.com**]. Our studies and those of other researchers have shown this step counter to be the most accurate; it costs from $15 to $25.)

Step counters look a lot like electronic pagers. They contain a small pendulum that moves each time the wearer takes a step. For the greatest accuracy it is important to keep the step counter centered over the left hipbone, lined up with the front crease of the wearer's slacks. The step counter *must* be firmly attached, so it is best worn on a belt or attached to the waistband of exercise shorts, pants, or undergarments. If your client chooses to wear the step counter on her underwear or pantyhose, she should put it inside not outside the waistband. Also, she should be sure to remove the step counter before using the bathroom.

Advise your client to put on the step counter first thing in the morning and keep it on until bedtime. When he takes it off at bedtime, he should record the number of steps he took that day. A sample log sheet (figure 7.6) is provided on page 105 at the end of this chapter. Next he should reset the step counter back to zero for the next day of use.

In the studies with which we are familiar (e.g., Welk, Differding, Thompson, Blair, Dziura, & Hart, 2000), most people accumulate 2,000 to 4,000 steps per day while performing their daily routines (walking around the house or office, doing daily chores, getting in and out of the car on errands, and the like). Walking for 30 minutes at a brisk pace equals about 4,000 steps. These numbers can help you and your client to set realistic short- and long-term goals. Other steps are accumulated through more activity in daily life, such as parking and walking into a fast food restaurant rather than using the drive through, parking at the far end of a shopping mall parking lot, and so on. Also, data show that people who are meeting the national guidelines tend to average 10,000 steps or more (Welk et al., 2000).

After your client has recorded her steps for a week, her average steps per day can be calculated. Then you can help her set a reasonable goal and devise a plan for increasing her steps to reach that goal. The long-term goal we usually recommend is 10,000 steps a day, because this has been shown to be enough to obtain important health benefits (Welk et al., 2000). However, for a client who is taking only 2,500 steps per day, you may *not* want to talk with her about a long-term goal of obtaining 10,000 steps per day. Rather, you may want to set a goal of 5,000 steps per day, which is more easily attainable for a person at that activity level. Once this goal is realized, you and your client can reevaluate and set the next goal. You may want to create a form for your client to track progress over time. A simple graph that you or your client fills out can be a useful way to demonstrate that your client has made great progress or has lots of room to improve.

Step counters can help your clients stay on track. You may want to instruct them to regularly check to see how many steps they have taken. If it's already midafternoon and a client has accumulated only 1,500 steps, he needs to find a way to get in a lot more activity that day. He may need to think creatively about how to get in some purposeful activity, such as taking a 20-minute walk home from the commuter rail station rather than getting a ride with a neighbor or taking a 10-minute walk rather than a coffee break in the afternoon.

Fitness Assessment

We have described means for measuring your clients' physical activity and patterns of behavior. Understanding these patterns is critical to helping your clients see more benefits and fewer barriers to living an active lifestyle and to enhancing your clients' motivation to become more physically active. However, your clients' actual physical fitness is also an important factor in increasing their levels of physical activity. If a client has a very high resting heart rate and cannot walk even half a mile (0.8 kilometers) without becoming breathless, he needs to start an activity program very slowly, even if he is extremely motivated to change. For example, this client could start off performing 2-minute bouts of activity and then slowly move up to 5- and then 10-minute bouts. On the other hand, if your client is fit enough to easily accomplish a half-mile walk but feels that she is too busy to be active, your physical activity plan may focus more on rearranging her schedule. You can encourage this client to turn light activity into moderate-intensity activity and to string short bouts of activity together into longer bouts of activity without necessarily adding to your client's busy day. Activity pattern assessment and physical fitness assessment work hand in hand to help you to customize a program that will best meet your client's needs and that she can start and stick with, thereby enhancing the likelihood that she will eventually be regularly active on a daily basis.

Resting Heart Rate

One of the simplest ways to gauge changes in fitness is to track the resting heart rate (beats per minute). As a client's fitness improves, his resting heart rate slows down. This happens because when a person exercises, the heart gets stronger and can pump more blood with each beat than when he is inactive.

Your clients may not know how to measure their resting heart rate. The easiest place to find a pulse is the inside of the wrist, just below the thumb. Help your clients learn how to place the index and middle fingers lightly against the artery at that location. A client may need to move her fingers around a bit until she is able to feel the rhythmic beat of her pulse (figure 7.3). Next, using a second hand on a watch or a stopwatch, have her count how many times her heart beats in one minute. Then she can record it on a form like the one shown in figure 7.7 on page 105 of this chapter. To ensure the accuracy of this measure, advise your client to take her heart rate first thing in the morning, when she has not yet had any coffee or cigarettes, as either of these stimulants could greatly affect her resting heart rate.

Depending on your situation and your plans for working with your client, you rather than your client can do the measurement and recording. If you are working with an individual who has numerous risk factors for

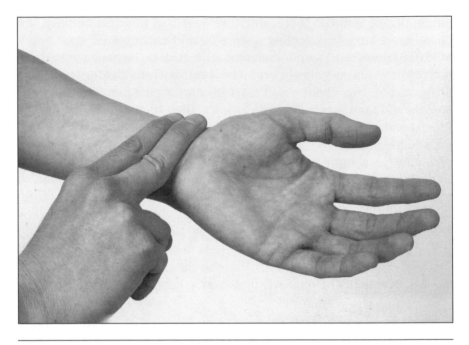

Figure 7.3 Taking a pulse by palpation.

heart disease and has repeatedly tried but failed to become more active, you may want to be more proactive. However, if you are working with a more motivated individual who wants to work with you only briefly and then work more independently, it is probably best to give him more autonomy from the beginning and teach him how to record his heart rate on his own.

Every month (or whatever interval makes sense in your situation) have your client measure and record her resting heart rate. If she is regularly participating in physical activity, her resting heart rate should decrease over time. Depending on the circumstances, you may also want your client to record whether or not she is experiencing any extreme emotions such as stress, worry, or sadness. Strong emotional responses can affect heart rate and may help you to interpret unexpected patterns in her heart rate over time.

Walking Test

A simple and inexpensive way to assess changes in fitness is a walking test. Your client needs access to a one-half-mile (0.8-kilometer) track or to map out his own half-mile route. Alternatively, you can suggest a route near the facility where you work with this client. Be sure your client warms up first by walking slowly for a few minutes. Then you can time him, or have him time himself, as he walks this route as quickly as possible. In some settings, it may be efficient for a group of individuals or employees to perform this test at the same time. You or your client should record how long it took to walk the half mile and also his heart rate immediately after he finishes the half mile so that you can determine how hard he was working while he walked that distance (figure 7.8 on page 106 of this chapter). Advise your client to refrain from cigarette smoking and coffee and cola consumption for at least one hour prior to this walking test because these stimulants can raise the heart rate. The client should repeat this test every couple of months to determine progress.

Assessing Physical Activity and Fitness in Group Settings

All of the methods for measuring physical activity patterns and physical fitness described in this chapter can be used in settings involving more than one client at a time. Instructions for filling out the forms for determining physical activity habits can be given to a group; then people can complete them individually, and you can provide individual feedback to each. If you work with too many people for you to meet with each individually, you may be able to provide feedback to small groups who are confronting similar issues, depending on the confidentiality requirements in your setting.

Another way to use these materials might be to put detailed instructions and forms on a Web site that is password protected (to maintain privacy and confidentiality) and available only to your clients. This allows you to provide individualized feedback and answers to questions via e-mail, a chat room, or an electronic bulletin board.

The physical fitness assessments can also be administered to a group. Similarly, a Web site can be used to provide clients with various one-half-mile walking routes in their local areas as well as the tracking forms to record and track their changes over time.

CONCLUSION

In this chapter we explained why it is important to understand and track your client's physical activity patterns and physical fitness and provided you with the strategies we think will be most helpful in accomplishing these objectives. We provided tools for tracking your client's activity habits because tracking these habits is critical in helping your client to come up with realistic, measurable goals for change. We also described how to use the methods presented in this chapter with more than one client at a time. Now that you are familiar with assessment methods, you are ready to learn about applying the stages-of-change model in your work with clients.

Activity	Intensity level	10-minute bouts	30-minute bouts	Total minutes
Housework	Light			
	Moderate/vigorous			
Occupation	Light			
	Moderate/vigorous			
Leisure	Light			
	Moderate/vigorous			
Gardening	Light			
	Moderate/vigorous			
Sports	Light			
	Moderate/vigorous			
Walking	Light			
	Moderate/vigorous			
Stairs	Light			
	Moderate/vigorous			

Figure 7.4 Blank activity-tracking sheet.

From *Motivating People to Be Physically Active*, by Bess H. Marcus and LeighAnn H. Forsyth, 2003, Human Kinetics, Champaign, IL.

Date: _____ Day of week: _____

Time slot	Activities, chores, errands, work, child care, leisure	Physically active? Yes	No
7:00 A.M. to 9:00 A.M.			
9:00 A.M. to 11:00 A.M.			
11:00 A.M. to 1:00 P.M.			
1:00 P.M. to 3:00 P.M.			
3:00 P.M. to 5:00 P.M.			
5:00 P.M. to 7:00 P.M.			

(continued)

Figure 7.5 Time-tracking sheet.

Time slot	Activities, chores, errands, work, child care, leisure	Physically active? Yes	No
7:00 P.M. to 9:00 P.M.			
9:00 P.M. to 11:00 P.M			
11:00 P.M. to 1:00 A.M			
1:00 A.M. to 3:00 A.M			
3:00 A.M. to 5:00 A.M			
5:00 A.M. to 7:00 A.M			

Figure 7.5 *(continued)*

Week: _____

Day of week	Date	Step goal	Actual steps	Minutes of activity	Notes
Sunday					
Monday					
Tuesday					
Wednesday					
Thursday					
Friday					
Saturday					

Figure 7.6 Step-counter log.

Reprinted, by permission, from S.N. Blair et al., 2001, *Active Living Every Day* (Champaign, IL: Human Kinetics), 49.

Date	Resting heart rate

Figure 7.7 Resting heart rate log.

Date	Time to walk half mile (minutes and seconds)	Heart rate at end

Figure 7.8   Walking-test log.

Reprinted, by permission, from S.N. Blair et al., 2001, *Active Living Every Day* (Champaign, IL: Human Kinetics), 120.

References

A collection of physical activity questionnaires for health-related research. (1997). *Medicine and Science in Sports and Exercise, 29*(Suppl. 6).

Marcus, B.H., & Simkin, L.R. (1993). The stages of exercise behavior. *Journal of Sports Medicine and Physical Fitness, 33,* 83–88.

Measurement of physical activity [Special issue]. (2000). *Research Quarterly for Exercise and Sport, 71.*

Welk, G.J., Differding, J.A., Thompson, R.W., Blair, S.N., Dziura, J., & Hart, P. (2000). The utility of the Digi-Walker step counter to assess daily physical activity patterns. *Medicine and Science in Sports and Exercise 32*(9): S481–S488.

EIGHT

Using the Stages Model in Individual Counseling

The stages of motivational readiness for change model was originally developed to better understand how individuals change behavior on their own. The goal of studying how people change on their own was to discover the key ingredients in behavior change so that counselors and therapists could use these ingredients with individuals who want to change their behavior but are either unwilling or unable to do so on their own. This chapter on applying the stages-of-change model focuses on individual counseling.

We describe how to assess your client's physical readiness as well as psychological readiness to start a program of physical activity. We explain why it is important to examine your client's past experiences with changing habits and how to help your client solve problems that may be getting in the way of becoming more active. We also describe strategies for enhancing your client's confidence that she can successfully change her behavior and how to help her set realistic goals for behavior change. Each of these issues is pertinent at all stages of motivational readiness due to the cyclical nature of behavior change. Therefore, many of the areas described in this chapter need to be addressed repeatedly during initiation, adoption, and maintenance of a habit. However, these topics are addressed slightly differently for people at each stage. The Stage-Specific Strategies section at the end of this chapter (p. 119) provides some ideas for how you can apply each topic at each stage of motivational readiness when working with individuals. One of the first steps in individual counseling is to assess the client's motivational readiness for physical activity and to keep this in mind as you work with her using the strategies discussed in this chapter.

Physical Readiness

In chapter 1 we described the numerous health benefits of an active lifestyle. Although most people benefit from participating in a program of regular physical activity, those with health problems may need more medical supervision than you or your facility can provide. Thus, it is important to first assess your client's physical readiness for physical activity before embarking on specific physical activity counseling with your client.

Depending on your professional training, you may or may not feel comfortable addressing the issue of safety with your client. In general, exercising at a moderate intensity (as opposed to vigorously) is safe for most people. For most people, a medical exam or stress test is not required before increasing moderate-intensity physical activities. Nevertheless, people who have diseases such as heart disease and diabetes should check with their doctors before beginning to exercise even at a moderate intensity. One often-used method of determining whether it is safe for a given person to increase his activity is the Physical Activity Readiness Questionnaire (PAR-Q; figure 8.1). Your client should read the questionnaire carefully and answer each yes-or-no question honestly.

If your client answers yes to one or more questions, she should speak with her doctor before she increases her physical activity. She should be sure to tell her doctor the specific questions to which she answered yes.

If your client answers no to all the questions, he can begin activity slowly and increase it gradually; it is your job to tell him how to do this. If you will work with this client for more than six months, you can periodically re-administer this questionnaire and have your client contact his doctor if he answers yes to any of the questions.

Because your client has come to you, chances are your client is pretty sedentary and should begin with moderate-intensity activities. However, if your client wants to exercise at a vigorous level, your client should check with a doctor first if one of the following applies:

1. your client is a man 45 or older or a woman 55 or older;
2. your client has *two* or more of the following risk factors: has a family history of heart disease, is a current cigarette smoker, has high blood pressure, has high cholesterol, has high blood sugar, is 30 pounds overweight or more, or is currently not at all active; *or*
3. your client has heart or blood vessel disease, diabetes, lung disease, asthma, thyroid disorder, or kidney disease.

Psychological Readiness

Physical readiness is not likely to be the main barrier to activity for most of your clients; rather, it is their psychological readiness for change. While you might not see a lot of stage 1 people in the setting in which you work, chances are good that you see lots of stage 2 clients, who keep meaning to start some physical activity but never get around to it. You may also see people in stage 3, who do some physical activity but have not quite figured out how to make it a habit of sufficient frequency

Physical Activity Readiness
Questionnaire – PAR-Q
(revised 1994)

PAR - Q & YOU

(A Questionnaire for People Aged 15 to 69)

Regular physical activity is fun and healthy, and increasingly more people are starting to become more active every day. Being more active is very safe for most people. However, some people should check with their doctor before they start becoming much more physically active.

If you are planning to become much more physically active than you are now, start by answering the seven questions in the box below. If you are between the ages of 15 and 69, the PAR-Q will tell you if you should check with your doctor before you start. If you are over 69 years of age, and you are not used to being very active, check with your doctor.

Common sense is your best guide when you answer these questions. Please read the questions carefully and answer each one honestly: check YES or NO.

YES	NO		
☐	☐	1.	Has your doctor ever said that you have a heart condition <u>and</u> that you should only do physical activity recommended by a doctor?
☐	☐	2.	Do you feel pain in your chest when you do physical activity?
☐	☐	3.	In the past month, have you had chest pain when you were not doing physical activity?
☐	☐	4.	Do you lose your balance because of dizziness or do you ever lose consciousness?
☐	☐	5.	Do you have a bone or joint problem that could be made worse by a change in your physical activity?
☐	☐	6.	Is your doctor currently prescribing drugs (for example, water pills) for your blood pressure or heart condition?
☐	☐	7.	Do you know of <u>any other reason</u> why you should not do physical activity?

If

you

answered

YES to one or more questions

Talk with your doctor by phone or in person BEFORE you start becoming much more physically active or BEFORE you have a fitness appraisal. Tell your doctor about the PAR-Q and which questions you answered YES.

- You may be able to do any activity you want—as long as you start slowly and build up gradually. Or, you may need to restrict your activities to those which are safe for you. Talk with your doctor about the kinds of activities you wish to participate in and follow his/her advice.
- Find out which community programs are safe and helpful for you.

NO to all questions

If you answered NO honestly to <u>all</u> PAR-Q questions, you can be reasonably sure that you can:

- start becoming much more physically active—begin slowly and build up gradually. This is the safest and easiest way to go.
- take part in a fitness appraisal—this is an excellent way to determine your basic fitness so that you can plan the best way for you to live actively.

DELAY BECOMING MUCH MORE ACTIVE:
- if you are not feeling well because of a temporary illness such as a cold or a fever—wait until you feel better; or
- if you are or may be pregnant—talk to your doctor before you start becoming more active.

Please note: If your health changes so that you then answer YES to any of the above questions, tell your fitness or health professional. Ask whether you should change your physical activity plan.

<u>Informed Use of the PAR-Q:</u> The Canadian Society for Exercise Physiology, Health Canada, and their agents assume no liability for persons who undertake physical activity, and if in doubt after completing this questionnaire, consult your doctor prior to physical activity.

You are encouraged to copy the PAR-Q but only if you use the entire form

NOTE: If the PAR-Q is being given to a person before he or she participates in a physical activity program or a fitness appraisal, this section may be used for legal or administrative purposes.

I have read, understood and completed this questionnaire. Any questions I had were answered to my full satisfaction.

NAME _____

SIGNATURE _____ DATE _____

SIGNATURE OF PARENT _____ WITNESS _____
or GUARDIAN (for participants under the age of majority)

©Canadian Society for Exercise Physiology   Supported by: Health   Santé
Société canadienne de physiologie de l'exercice   CANADA   Canada Canada

Figure 8.1 The physical activity readiness questionnaire.

Reprinted from the 1994 revised version of the Physical Activity Readiness Questionnaire (PAR-Q and YOU). The PAR-Q and YOU is a copyrighted, pre-exercise screen owned by the Canadian Society for Exercise Physiology.

and duration to obtain important health benefits. Your task with all your clients is to aid them in moving through the stages of change and helping them avoid pitfalls on what can be an arduous journey. You must help them understand how their behavior regarding physical activity is like other behaviors they have succeeded in changing in the past. You should help them examine the benefits and barriers to changing their behavior. You must assist them in solving problems that arise when they try to change their physical activity habits. You also need to aid them in building confidence in themselves and in setting realistic goals that they can achieve and thereby feel proud and successful.

Personal Successes and Past Behavior Change

Some clients may desire to become more active but tell you that they do not think they can succeed and that it seems overwhelming to think of changing their whole life around to become more active. One very effective tool for working with clients like these is to sidestep the issue of physical activity initially. Instead, start off by helping them to recall some other lifestyle change that they chose to make, with or without professional help, and at which they were successful. This is key because past behavior is the single strongest predictor of future behavior. Helping your client recall a past success is likely to empower her and catalyze her to make positive changes in her physical activity habits.

Have your client take a few minutes to relate one or more of her previous success stories: a healthy habit she has adopted or an unhealthy habit she has stopped. Then have her think about why she was able to make a successful change. What helped her succeed? What got in her way? For example, if your client successfully quit smoking by setting her 40th birthday as her quit date and receiving support from family, friends, and co-workers, this gives you and your client a lot of information about what might help her start a program of regular physical activity. Figure 8.2 on page 134 of this chapter is an example of a form you and your client might use to record these successes.

Once you and your client have discussed these successes and how they were achieved, you should have a lot of useful information about the strategies that work and do not work for your client. This information can help you to work with your client's areas of strength (e.g., a lot of supportive friends) and deal with areas of weakness or difficulty (e.g., a very stressful work environment). In this way you can create a program that is uniquely suited for your client and thus extremely likely to help your client succeed with his goals. For example, you may learn that when your client took a Thursday and Friday off from work and spent Thursday, Friday, Saturday, and Sunday surrounded by supportive friends and away from his stressful job, he was able to radically decrease the amount of coffee he consumed. This was a personal goal because his primary-care physician told him that decreased caffeine consumption might help decrease the frequency and intensity of his headaches. By the time your client returned to work the next Monday, he felt that he had established a new habit of making every other cup of coffee be decaffeinated. He was able to maintain this new habit with phone calls and e-mail from supportive friends over the next two weeks. This information about your client's past provides many important clues for helping him change his physical activity behavior. Where are those friends now? How can you help him to mobilize them? Can he take a couple of days off of work, or can he take 60 rather than 30 minutes for lunch so that he can fit in some physical activity?

Readiness to Change Physical Activity Habits

Some people believe that an individual just needs to make up her mind to do something and then she can do it, relying on a lot of willpower in the process. However, most behavior change happens slowly, and lasting behavior change occurs only when a person is motivated for change. Although some people can make major lifestyle changes on their own, many others need help—often from a person like you.

How does an individual know if he is ready to make a change? There are a number of ways to determine one's readiness for change. One way is for your client to ask himself the question, "What will I get as a result of making this behavior change?" (i.e., what are the benefits of change?). If your client cannot come up with at least a few key benefits, it is unlikely that your client will be able to accomplish even short-term change at this point in time. It's a good idea to have your client take a few moments to write down his reasons for wanting to change his activity habits. This exercise is useful for clients at all stages (even stage 1 people can list lots of reasons to become more active—they just have not acted on them) of motivational readiness because understanding the benefits of exercise is critical for taking up and sticking with a physically active lifestyle.

Another important component to changing behavior is determining what your client will have to give up or what she will find unpleasant if she makes a change. It is unrealistic to think that a person can make a major life transition such as becoming regularly active from being primarily inactive without having some aspects of the process be annoying or frustrating. Barriers to behavior change might get in the way of your client's best-laid plans. For example, if your client is worried that her family will feel burdened or neglected due to her physical activity, this key topic is something you should discuss with her. Have your client take a few minutes to generate a list of her barriers to physical activity behavior change. Sample forms for listing both benefits and barriers (figures 8.3 and 8.4) are on page 135 of this chapter.

Look over these lists with your client and examine the number and nature of the barriers. Work with your client to determine which are true barriers and which are excuses. For example, not walking after work because it is dark and the neighborhood is unsafe is a legitimate barrier to physical activity. However, preferring to spend leisure time shopping rather than being active is an excuse to not exercise. Work on problem-solving exercises to address the true barriers. The reason to focus on barriers is that, with your help, they can be removed. You can teach your client how to find more time in his day. You can guide your client in turning light activity into moderate-intensity activity. However, when you work with your client on modifying excuses, he may well come up with more excuses, and you can thus end up in a cyclical conversation that leaves you both frustrated. One strategy for problem solving is described in the next section.

The IDEA Approach to Problem Solving

Once your client identifies her barriers, the next step is to help her use some simple problem-solving skills. Problem solving means thinking creatively about the most effective solution to use when a problem gets in the way. Thinking creatively is key. It is important to encourage your client to be as creative as possible when coming up with solutions. Sometimes the most absurd solution actually works best! Once your client has come up with a variety of possible solutions, you need to help her choose one to try out first and later determine how well it worked. It is very important that you encourage your client to pick a good time to implement the solutions to enhance the likelihood of success. Also, you must help your client recognize that finding out that one solution does not work is not bad news. This information can help you find a solution that not only works but that can be maintained over time.

The IDEA technique is a simple problem-solving approach that has worked well in a number of our studies and with a number of our clients. It is easy to implement and can be helpful to all clients, especially those clients who are "stuck" by their barriers to behavior change. The goal is to help your client figuratively see the light bulb of a new option to help pull him out of his current situation and help him to emerge into the new situation he says he wants yet has been unable to attain.

Identify the Problem

First, have your client select one barrier and write it down on the IDEA form in figure 8.5 on page 136. Have your client think about how this barrier specifically keeps her from being active. Next, have your client write down the most important details about this personal barrier. For example, if your client's barrier is frequent business travel, she may say that she is concerned specifically about her personal safety when she is away from home.

Develop a List of Solutions

Help your client to brainstorm and come up with as many creative solutions as possible. If your client has trouble thinking up solutions, step in and offer some. Be sure to think broadly about possible options, and be sure to think carefully about what your client has already revealed to you when coming up with options. That is, try to personalize your responses as much as possible. Encourage your client not to worry about whether the solutions are good or bad, workable or unrealistic. That can come later. Sometimes a client's seemingly far-fetched ideas turn out to be the best solution. Write down all the ideas that come up, and encourage your client to keep the list with her for a few days and to add more solutions as she thinks of them.

Evaluate the Solutions

Some solutions seem more realistic than others. However, some solutions that seem far-fetched at first may appear more realistic with more thought. Work with your client to select one solution that she is willing to try. Then help your client to plan how and when to put it into action. For example, if your client's main barrier is business travel and the specific problem is that she does not feel safe and comfortable walking in an unfamiliar area, one solution could be to check ahead to make sure the hotel has an exercise facility and if it does not to switch hotels, if possible, to one that does have such a facility. Another plan might involve teaching her a set of simple aerobic exercises or a rope-jumping routine that she can take on the road and do in the safety of her hotel room. A third strategy might be to have her walk as much as she can while at the airport and in other heavily traveled areas where she feels safe.

Analyze How Well Your Plan Worked

After your client has given her plan a try, help her to analyze how well it worked. Help her to honestly examine what did and did not work. Then help her to revise her plan before she tries it again. For example, if your client is going to rely on a hotel exercise facility but does not get around to calling the hotel ahead of time and then finds that a facility is not available, it will be clear that her plan did not work because it was not fully implemented. Thus, there is no reason to throw this plan away; rather, it should be tried again. However, if she calls ahead to discover that there is an exercise facility, yet it is so crowded from 6 to 8 A.M. that she cannot exercise before her hectic 9 A.M. to 10 P.M. working day starts, then it might be necessary to revise the plan and perhaps try the rope-jumping routine the next time. Because most clients have more than one barrier to address, you can encourage them to use the IDEA form for other barriers once they have used it successfully.

Confidence Is Critical for Behavior Change

Having confidence in oneself is critical during all phases of behavior change. Years of research in the field of psychology demonstrate that assisting your client to believe in himself and visualize himself as someone who is or one day will be successful is paramount to helping him think about change, make change, and sustain this change over the years. Your job is really twofold. First, you need to regularly convey your belief that your client can and will succeed in his efforts to start or stick with a physical activity plan. Second, you need to teach your client the skills to believe in himself, as this is critical once his contact with you has concluded.

To gauge your client's level of confidence, you can ask him to rate his confidence that he can start or continue to be regularly physically active on a scale of 1 to 5, with the lowest level of confidence being 1 and the highest level 5. (For a more detailed questionnaire to measure confidence, see chapter 5.)

If your client answers 1 or 2, help your client think about why he does not feel confident, and discuss ways to help him become more confident. Pinpointing specific obstacles is often the first step to overcoming them. For example, if your client lacks confidence that he can exercise after work due to family responsibilities, you can work with him at enhancing his confidence that he can walk during breaks and lunch time and thus have already accumulated 30 minutes of physical activity before he goes home.

If your client rates his confidence a 3, your client is halfway there. Help your client to think about what he likes most and least about physical activity. Do what you can to help make physical activity more enjoyable, convenient, or safe for your client. For example, you can discuss whether your client prefers to be active alone or with others and whether he prefers to be active during the workday or before or after work. You can examine why your client has these preferences. Perhaps your client prefers walking alone because he is embarrassed that he is too unfit to jog, the activity in which many of his friends participate. This may be important information if you learn that your client actually prefers being active with others and aspires to join his friends eventually for early morning jogs.

If your client answered 4 or 5, your client is well on his way to making exercise a lifelong habit. Maintaining a physically active lifestyle is extremely challenging. Staying active requires continued time, energy, and planning for a lifetime. To stay regularly active, a person needs to set the alarm clock to go off early in the morning or skip part of lunch to take a walk or stop at the gym on the way home from work every day. Participating in physical activity never ceases to be an issue. Your client may well begin to truly enjoy activity and even look forward to it. However, it always takes thought, time, and planning. Thus, it is critical that your client keep up his confidence that he can stick with physical activity even during difficult times of stress, sadness, extreme pressure at work, and the like. It is also important that you work with your client to instill the confidence that he can start up his physical activity program anew if his efforts get derailed for some reason, such as following the birth of his first child or relocation to a new city.

Setting Goals

You must help your client figure out what her goals are; otherwise, it will be very difficult for you to help her with her activity plan. The goals you set together become the contract you two agree to pursue. For example, if your client's goal is weight loss, her short-term goal may be walking daily for 15 minutes, a medium-term goal may be walking daily for 30 minutes, and her long-term goal may be walking daily for 60 minutes. Your role is to help your client achieve those goals. Additionally, the clearer the goals that your client sets, the better her chances of reaching these goals. Teaching your client effective ways of setting goals can go a long way toward helping her succeed. Figure 8.6 (page 137 of this chapter) is an example of a form that you and your client can use to record goals. Here are three important tips for goal setting:

- **Be specific.** People who set specific goals do better than people who say only, "I'll try to do my best." For example, if your client says, "This week I'll try to be more active," help him to turn this into a specific goal such as, "This week I'll walk for 15 minutes every lunch hour and another 15 minutes after dinner." Specific goals tend to be effective because they are measurable. Also, with your assistance, these specific goals should be ones that are attainable by your client. Goal setting is related to confidence building; if your client reaches a goal he has set, he will have increased confidence that he can progress to meet his next goal.

- **Set both short-term and long-term goals.** If your client's goal is to walk an hour a day, five days a week, you need to help her not to expect to reach that goal immediately. You need to assist her in recognizing the need to start off slowly yet never to lose sight of the goal. A good short-term goal might be to walk for three 10-minute bouts each on Sunday, Wednesday, and Friday, then gradually increase the number of minutes and the number of days a week that she walks. In this way, you help her build confidence that she can meet the goals she sets, which can then empower her to set future goals. Reaching the goal one sets creates a sense of mastery and a warm sense of achievement. Nothing is more important in helping your client attain and maintain her long-term goals.

- **Give your client feedback, and teach him to give himself feedback.** Choose a way to track your client's progress. Assessment tools are suggested in chapters 2, 5, and 7. Monitoring progress lets your

117

client see the pattern of ups and downs and helps him understand that the downs are only temporary. He can then learn strategies to turn these downs into ups and to avoid some of these downs in the future.

Measuring Success

There are several ways to measure success in physical activity. You could help your client to add up the time she spends doing an activity and to set a goal for increasing her activity time. Alternatively, you can measure success by using any of the questionnaires provided in chapters 2 and 5. These questionnaires can be re-administered every three months, and you and your client can evaluate the new strategies she has learned and other strategies that may be helpful for her short- and long-term success.

Goal setting is valuable only when there is a way to measure success in attaining goals. For your client to feel successful, it is important to agree on a means for measuring success. At different points in time, you may measure success by different means. Initially, success may be measured more by changes in the mediators of change in physical activity described in chapters 4 and 5. Later, success may be measured by forward progression in the stages of change as described in chapter 2 or by changes in fitness as described in chapter 7. Measuring success is important for keeping your client on track and ensuring that short- and long-term goals stay realistic.

Stage-Specific Strategies for Individual Counseling

This section provides some guidelines, suggestions, and ideas for you to use in individual counseling with your clients. More importantly, these strategies are broken down in a stage-specific format for ease of use.

STAGE 1

Not Thinking About Change

Even though your client is not considering becoming physically active right now, you still can do some brief counseling to help your client move toward thinking about behavior change. Here are some ways you can apply each of the strategies discussed in the chapter for a client in this earliest stage.

Is your client physically ready to consider physical activity?

- Give your client the PAR-Q (figure 8.1) to identify any health reasons for not considering physical activity.
- Discuss moderate-intensity activity as less likely to cause adverse health events.
- Refer your client to a physician if any health problems exist.

How has your client successfully changed behavior in the past?

- Increase your client's confidence by discussing her past attempts at behavior change and identifying strategies that worked then and could help with physical activity change in the future.
- Resolve problematic strategies that have gotten in the way during past attempts at behavior change.

How might your client benefit from physical activity?

- Ask your client to write down how she might benefit from some physical activity.
- Suggest some benefits your client may not have thought of yet.
- Encourage your client to read and learn more about benefits.
- Have your client assess how important these benefits are for her.

What might your client need to give up to become physically active, and what barriers does your client need to address?

- Ask your client to write down what she would have to give up to become physically active and what she might find unpleasant about physical activity.
- Have your client assess how important these issues are to her.
- Help your client to differentiate between true barriers and excuses.
- Begin to find solutions to these barriers using the IDEA approach.

How can you help your client to become more confident about physical activity?

- Let your client know that you believe in her ability to become a physically active individual someday.

(continued)

(continued)

- Reinforce any action your client takes that can help her think about trying some physical activity (e.g., talking to others about physical activity, reading about it, thinking about how she might benefit if she were to become physically active).
- Ask your client to assess her confidence in someday becoming more active on a scale from 1 (not confident) to 5 (very confident).
- Work on increasing your client's confidence by trying to pinpoint perceived obstacles and developing realistic strategies for overcoming them.
- Relate your client's past successes at behavior change with her ability to become physically active in the future.
- Discuss what went wrong during past attempts at behavior change and reframe them as learning experiences that can teach your client what to do differently should she decide to become physically active.

What goals might help your client move toward behavior change?

- Work with your client to set a manageable, short-term goal, perhaps around a mediator of behavior change that can help your client to start thinking about changing her sedentary lifestyle.
- Your client can discuss with her physician how she might personally benefit from some physical activity (comprehending benefits).
- Another short-term goal might be to have your client use the IDEA approach on her own to work out a possible solution for one or two of her perceived barriers (decisional balance).
- Ask your client to try to spot a person similar to herself in age, body shape, health status, and so on who is being physically active (self-efficacy).
- Have your client ask a friend or family member to take over child care or household responsibilities for an hour so that she can spend some time reading about physical activity or touring a local facility (enlisting social support, increasing knowledge).
- Ask your client to write down some ways that her sedentary lifestyle is affecting people important to her (caring about consequences to others).
- Agree on something your client can do or a small gift she can buy herself to reward success in achieving this goal (rewarding oneself).
- Suggest that your client allow herself to engage in a pleasurable sedentary activity (e.g., watching a favorite movie, surfing the Web, taking a short nap) only after she has accomplished one of the preceding goals.

- Set up a point system that your client can use to earn a larger reward (e.g., accomplishing a small goal can earn 2 points; 20 accumulated points can be used to "purchase" a night at the movies or some personal time).
- Reinforce the idea that achieving other behavioral or cognitive goals, even if they do not include actual physical activity, are productive and worthwhile.

How can you measure your client's success?

- Reassess your client's stage of change.
- Consider giving your client the processes-of-change questionnaire in chapter 5 on page 61 to see whether she is using more strategies.
- Measure your client's confidence to see whether it has improved by using the self-efficacy questionnaire in chapter 5 (page 65).
- Reassess perceived benefits relative to perceived barriers using the decisional balance questionnaire in chapter 5 on page 67.
- Ask your client to simply rate how satisfied she is with her progress on a 1–5 scale.

STAGE 2

Thinking About Change

Your client is thinking about becoming more active, so your task is to help her commit to a start date and do some planning that will enhance the likelihood that she will be successful in this endeavor and find her physical activity experience pleasant enough to try it again. Here are some ideas for helping a client who is thinking about change but has not engaged in any actual physical activity.

Is your client physically ready to begin physical activity?

- Give your client the PAR-Q (figure 8.1) to identify any health reasons for not starting some physical activity.
- Discuss moderate-intensity activity as less likely to cause adverse health events.
- Refer your client to a physician if any health problems exist or if your client expresses interest in starting with vigorous activity.

How has your client successfully changed behavior in the past?

- Increase your client's self-efficacy by discussing his past attempts at behavior change and identifying strategies that worked then and could help with beginning physical activity.
- Resolve problematic strategies that have gotten in the way during past attempts at behavior change and may become an issue for changing physical activity habits.

How might your client benefit from becoming physically active?

- Ask your client to write down how he might benefit from physical activity.
- Suggest some benefits your client may not have thought of yet.
- Encourage your client to read and learn more about benefits.
- Have your client assess how important these benefits are to him.

What might your client need to give up to become physically active, and what barriers does your client need to address?

- Ask your client to write down what he would have to give up to become physically active and what he might find unpleasant about physical activity.
- Have your client assess how important these issues are to him.
- Help your client to differentiate between true barriers and excuses.
- Begin to find solutions to these barriers using the IDEA approach.

How can you help your client to become more confident about physical activity?

- Let your client know that you believe in his ability to become a physically active individual.
- Emphasize that your client has already made progress because he is thinking about becoming physically active.
- Work on increasing your client's confidence by trying to pinpoint perceived obstacles and developing realistic strategies for overcoming them.
- Relate your client's past successes at behavior change with his ability to become physically active in the future.
- Discuss what went wrong during past attempts at behavior change and reframe them as learning experiences that can teach your client what to do differently should he decide to become physically active.
- Begin to identify types of activities that might be manageable and also enjoyable for your client to try when he is ready. Plan when, where, and with whom your client might do this activity so that he can clearly visualize it taking place.

What goals might help your client move toward behavior change?

- Work with your client to set manageable short- and long-term goals, perhaps around a mediator of behavior change that can help your client to move closer to actually trying some physical activity.
- Recommend that your client make a few calls to learn where he might perform his chosen activity (increasing knowledge).
- Ask your client to try the IDEA approach on his own to work out possible solutions for one or two of the obstacles that seem to get in the way of actually trying some activity (decisional balance).
- Recommend that your client ask someone close to him to help solve some of the problems that are holding him back (enlisting social support).
- Suggest that your client commit himself to actually trying a brief, manageable bout of physical activity, such as a five-minute walk (self-efficacy; committing oneself).
- Ask your client to look up how many calories are burned for some of the activities he thinks he would be more likely to do (outcome expectations).
- Ask your client to complete a personal time study (e.g., monitoring time spent in sedentary pursuits and in physical activity for a typical week day and weekend day; increasing knowledge).

(continued)

123

(continued)

- Ask your client to write down some ways that his sedentary lifestyle is affecting people important to him (caring about consequences to others).
- Agree on something your client can do or a small gift he can buy himself to reward success in achieving these goals (rewarding oneself).
- Suggest that your client allow himself to engage in a pleasurable sedentary activity (e.g., watching a favorite movie, surfing the Web, taking a short nap) only after he has accomplished one of the preceding activity goals.
- Set up a point system that your client can use to earn a larger reward (e.g., accomplishing a small goal may earn 2 points; 20 accumulated points can be used to "purchase" a weekend at a bed-and-breakfast).
- Reinforce the idea that achieving goals, even if they do not include actual physical activity, are productive and worthwhile.

Has your client been successful in moving toward becoming physically active?

- Reassess your client's stage of change.
- Consider giving your client the processes-of-change questionnaire in chapter 5 on page 61.
- Measure your client's confidence by using the self-efficacy questionnaire in chapter 5 on page 65 to see whether it has improved.
- Reassess perceived benefits relative to perceived barriers using the decisional balance questionnaire on page 67.
- Ask your client to simply rate how satisfied he is with his progress on a 1–5 scale.

STAGE 3
Doing Some Physical Activity

Your client is doing some physical activity but not enough, so you need to help her develop some additional strategies for increasing her activity level. Here are some ideas for a client in this stage.

Is your client physically ready to increase physical activity?

- Give your client the PAR-Q (figure 8.1) to identify any health reasons for not increasing physical activity.
- Discuss moderate-intensity activity as less likely to cause adverse health events.
- Refer your client to a physician if any health problems exist or if your client expresses interest in starting to do vigorous-intensity activity and has one of the risk factors listed on page 109.

How has your client successfully changed behavior in the past?

- Increase your client's self-efficacy by discussing her past attempts at behavior change and identifying strategies that worked then and could help with increasing physical activity now.
- Resolve problematic strategies that have gotten in the way during past attempts at behavior change and may become an issue for changing physical activity.

How might your client benefit from increasing physical activity?

- Ask your client to write down how she might benefit from increasing her physical activity.
- Suggest some benefits your client may not have thought of yet or has not yet noticed.
- Encourage your client to read and learn more about these benefits and to look for additional benefits of increasing physical activity.
- Have your client assess how important these benefits are to her.

What might your client need to give up to become more physically active, and what barriers does your client need to address?

- Ask your client to write down what she would have to give up to increase physical activity and what she might find unpleasant about physical activity.
- Have your client assess how difficult these things will be to give up
- Help your client to differentiate between true barriers and excuses.
- Begin to find solutions for these barriers using the IDEA approach.

(continued)

(continued)

How can you help your client to become more confident about physical activity?

- Let your client know that you believe in her ability to increase her physical activity.

- Emphasize that your client has already made progress because she is doing some physical activity.

- Work on increasing your client's confidence by trying to pinpoint perceived obstacles and developing realistic strategies for overcoming them.

- Relate your client's past successes at behavior change with her ability to become more physically active.

- Discuss what went wrong during past attempts at behavior change and reframe them as learning experiences that can teach your client what to do differently this time around.

- Help your client to think about what she likes most and least about physical activity and how her activity plans can be modified to reflect these preferences.

- Encourage your client to think of herself as a physically active individual.

What goals might help your client become more physically active?

- Work with your client to set manageable, short- and long-term goals, perhaps around a mediator of behavior change that can help your client increase her physical activity.

- Create a plan for replacing 15 minutes of sedentary time during the week with some type of activity (substituting alternatives).

- Your client can set a goal of calling up a friend to join her for a 20-minute walk in the upcoming week (enlisting social support).

- Have your client think of a couple of ways to remind herself to be more active and try to implement them over the week (reminding oneself).

- Your client can commit herself to increasing her daily activity by five more minutes over the next week (self-efficacy; committing oneself).

- Agree on something your client can do or a small gift she can buy herself to reward success in achieving these goals (rewarding oneself).

- Suggest that your client allow herself to engage in a pleasurable sedentary activity (e.g., watching a favorite movie, surfing the Web, taking a short nap) only after she has accomplished one of the preceding activity goals.

- Set up a point system that your client can use to earn a larger reward (e.g., accomplishing a small goal may earn 2 points; 30 accumulated points can be used to "purchase" a camping trip).
- Discuss what someone significant in your client's life might be able to do or say to reward your client's physical activity achievements (enlisting social support).

Has your client been successful in increasing physical activity?

- Have your client keep a daily activity log to monitor minutes of activity.
- Ask your client to write down the number of steps accumulated on a pedometer over the course of the day.
- Reassess your client's stage of change.
- Consider giving your client the processes-of-change questionnaire in chapter 5 on page 61 to see whether she is using more strategies for change.
- Measure your client's confidence to see whether it has improved by using the self-efficacy questionnaire in chapter 5 on page 65.
- Administer the decisional balance questionnaire on page 67.

STAGE 4

Doing Enough Physical Activity

Even though your client is physically active at the recommended level, his challenge is to maintain his physical activity over time. Here are some suggestions for using the strategies discussed in this chapter to help a client in this stage to make physical activity a habit.

Is it physically safe for your client to continue being physically active?

- Give your client the PAR-Q (figure 8.1) to assess any changes in health status relevant to physical activity.
- Refer your client to a physician if any health problems or discomfort related to activity arises.

How has your client successfully changed behavior in the past?

- Discuss your client's past attempts at behavior change to identify strategies that he may not have yet applied to physical activity.
- Resolve problematic strategies that have gotten in the way during past attempts at behavior change and may be an issue for continuing physical activity.

How has your client benefited from becoming physically active?

- Ask your client to write down how he has benefited from his physical activity.
- Suggest some benefits your client may not have thought of yet or has not yet noticed.
- Encourage your client to read and learn more about benefits and to look for additional benefits as he continues to be physically active.
- Have your client assess how important these benefits are to him.

What are the costs of being physically active? What barriers might your client still need to address?

- Ask your client to write down what he has given up to become physically active and what he still finds unpleasant about physical activity.
- Have your client assess how important these things are to him.
- Use the IDEA problem-solving approach to reduce any perceived costs and any remaining barriers.
- Encourage your client to think about any obstacles that might arise in the future that could interfere with his ability to stay active. Create a plan for these potential problems.

How can your client become even more confident about physical activity?

- Discuss any negative thoughts concerning physical activity with which your client is still struggling and work on developing more positive thoughts.
- Help your client to think about what he likes most and least about physical activity. Find out what you can do to help make physical activity more enjoyable, convenient, or safe for your client.
- Work with your client to instill confidence that he can start up his physical activity program anew, if for some reason he should stop.
- Remind your client of how far he has come and praise him for his efforts.

What goals might help your client stay physically active?

- Help your client to generate short-term goals for physical activity or for mediators that may help him to sustain his motivation.
- Help your client to decide on an appropriate amount of activity in a given week (committing oneself).
- Suggest that your client try a new activity (enjoyment).
- Encourage your client to ask someone to exercise with him (enlisting social support).
- Suggest that your client think of someone in his life for whom he can serve as a role model. Have your client commit to a behavior that might help motivate this person to become active (caring about consequences to others, committing oneself).
- Be sure to help your client to develop some long-term goals (committing oneself).
- Find a walking or running event or race that is going to take place in the community. Work on a plan for your client to train for this event (committing oneself).
- Set up a reward plan for your client's continued regular activity for the next month (rewarding oneself).
- Help your client decide on a number of miles to try to accumulate over the next three months.
- Consult with a health professional if necessary to determine appropriate physiological goals for your client, such as decreasing cholesterol or blood pressure.
- Agree on a small gift your client can buy himself for accomplishing his goal (rewarding oneself).

(continued)

(continued)

- Suggest that your client allow himself to engage in a pleasurable sedentary activity (e.g., watching a favorite movie, surfing the Web, taking a short nap) only after he has accomplished one of the preceding activity goals.
- Set up a point system that your client can use to earn a larger reward (e.g., accomplishing a small goal may earn 2 points; 50 accumulated points can be used to "purchase" new walking shoes).
- Discuss what someone significant in your client's life might be able to do or say to reward your client's physical activity achievements (enlisting social support).
- Remind your client to review some of the benefits he has already achieved from physical activity. These benefits are natural rewards for exercising.
- Suggest that your client post some reminders in his environment so that he remembers to praise himself for his success (reminding oneself).

How can your client track success?

- Have your client keep a daily activity log to monitor minutes of activity.
- Ask your client to write down the number of steps accumulated on a pedometer over the course of the day. Develop a plan for your client to reward himself after he achieves a particular number.
- Suggest that your client monitor resting heart rate or level of exertion during activity. Record these on a graph that displays changes over time.
- If your client has a short period of inactivity (due to work demands, illness, etc.) but then resumes activity following this episode, praise him for his ability to get back on track.

STAGE 5

Making Physical Activity a Habit

Your client is somewhat of a seasoned pro if she is in this stage. However, you can be beneficial to her by using the strategies discussed in this chapter to help her prepare for any future setbacks and help her increase her enjoyment of physical activity:

Is it physically safe for your client to continue being physically active?

- Give your client the PAR-Q (figure 8.1) to assess any changes in health status relevant to physical activity.
- Refer your client to a physician if any health problems arise.

How has your client successfully changed behavior in the past?

- Discuss your client's past attempts at behavior change to identify strategies that she may not have applied yet to physical activity.
- Resolve problematic strategies that have gotten in the way during past attempts at behavior change and may be an issue for continuing physical activity.

How has your client benefited from continuing to be physically active?

- Suggest some benefits your client may not have noticed.
- Encourage your client to read and learn more about benefits.
- Encourage your client to periodically remind herself of how she benefits from continuing to be physically active; this helps to sustain motivation.

What are the costs of being physically active? What barriers might your client still need to address?

- Ask your client to write down what she has given up to become physically active and what she still finds unpleasant about physical activity.
- Have your client assess how important these things are to her.
- Use the IDEA problem-solving approach to further reduce any perceived costs.
- Work on ways to increase enjoyment.
- Encourage your client to think about any obstacles that might arise in the future that could interfere with her ability to stay active. Create a plan for these potential problems.

How can your client maintain confidence about staying active over the long term?

- Explore options for making activity more enjoyable.

(continued)

131

(continued)

- Work with your client to instill confidence that she can start up her physical activity program anew, if for some reason she should stop.
- Remind your client of how far she has come and praise her for her efforts.
- Remind your client of the benefits she has already achieved.
- Encourage your client to become a mentor to someone else who is trying to accomplish what she already has.

What goals might help your client stay physically active?

- Help your client to generate short-term goals that help to sustain her motivation (committing oneself).
- Suggest that your client try a new activity (enjoyment).
- Encourage your client to ask someone to be physically active with her (enlisting social support).
- Suggest that your client think of someone in her life for whom she can serve as a role model. Have your client commit to a behavior that might help motivate this person to become active (caring about consequences to others, committing oneself).
- Be sure to help your client to develop some long-term goals (committing oneself).
- Find a walking or running event or race that is going to take place in the community. Work on a plan for your client to train for this event (committing oneself).
- Set up a reward plan for your client's continued regular activity for the next month (rewarding oneself).
- Help your client decide on a number of miles to try to accumulate over the next three months (goal setting).
- Consult with a health professional if necessary to determine appropriate physiological goals for your client, such as decreasing cholesterol or blood pressure.
- Agree on a small gift your client can buy herself for accomplishing her goal (rewarding oneself).
- Suggest that your client allow herself to engage in some pleasurable activity (e.g., talking to a friend on the phone) only after she has accomplished one of the preceding activity goals.
- Set up a point system that your client can use to earn a larger reward (e.g., accomplishing a small goal may earn 2 points; 80 accumulated points can be used to "purchase" new exercise equipment).

- Discuss what someone significant in your client's life might be able to do or say to reward your client's physical activity achievements (enlisting social support).
- Remind your client to look over some of the benefits she has already achieved from physical activity. These benefits are natural rewards for exercising.
- Suggest that your client post some reminders in her environment so that she remembers to praise herself for her success (reminding oneself).

How can your client track success?

- Have your client keep a daily activity log to monitor minutes of activity.
- Ask your client to write down the number of steps accumulated on a pedometer over the course of the day. Help your client develop a plan for rewarding herself after she achieves a particular number.
- Suggest that your client monitor resting heart rate or level of exertion during activity. Have your client record these on a graph that displays changes over time.
- If your client has a short period of inactivity (due to work demands, illness, etc.) but then resumes activity following this episode, praise her for her ability to get back on track.

CONCLUSION

In this chapter we showed how the stages-of-change model can be applied when working with individuals. We shared the rationale and tools for assessing your client's physical and psychological readiness for physical activity. We also described the importance of your client's past experiences in making behavior changes and how this information can guide current plans for behavior change. Specific strategies for measuring your client's confidence and for goal setting were described. We also discussed the need to measure change in your client's behavior so as to empower her to continue the journey of behavior change and maintenance.

Habits I've changed
1.
2.
3.
Things that helped me succeed
1.
2.
3.
Obstacles that got in my way
1.
2.
3.

Figure 8.2 Record of past successes.

From *Motivating People to Be Physically Active,* by Bess H. Marcus and LeighAnn H. Forsyth, 2003, Human Kinetics, Champaign, IL.

Benefits of physical activity
1.
2.
3.
4.
5.
6.
7.
8.

Figure 8.3 Record of benefits of physical activity.

From *Motivating People to Be Physically Active,* by Bess H. Marcus and LeighAnn H. Forsyth, 2003, Human Kinetics, Champaign, IL.

Physical activity barriers
1.
2.
3.
4.
5.
6.
7.
8.

Figure 8.4 Record of physical activity barriers.

From *Motivating People to Be Physically Active,* by Bess H. Marcus and LeighAnn H. Forsyth, 2003, Human Kinetics, Champaign, IL.

Identify a barrier that keeps you from being active (or more active, or as active as you would like to be).

Develop a few creative solutions.

Evaluate your list of solutions. In the following space, write the solution you are willing to try and exactly *when* you will put it into action.

Analyze how well your plan worked and revise it if necessary. If your plan worked well, great! If your plan did not work too well, you will need to look back at your list of solutions and try again.

Figure 8.5   IDEA form.

Adapted, by permission, from S.N. Blair et al., 2001, *Active Living Every Day* (Champaign, IL: Human Kinetics), 31.

My short-term goal that I plan to achieve next week:

How I plan to monitor my progress on reaching this goal:

My long-term goal I plan to achieve by _____ **(date):**

How I plan to monitor my progress on reaching this goal:

Figure 8.6 Setting goals form.

Adapted, by permission, from S.N. Blair et al., 2001, *Active Living Every Day* (Champaign, IL: Human Kinetics), 31.

From *Motivating People to Be Physically Active,* by Bess H. Marcus
and LeighAnn H. Forsyth, 2003, Human Kinetics, Champaign, IL.

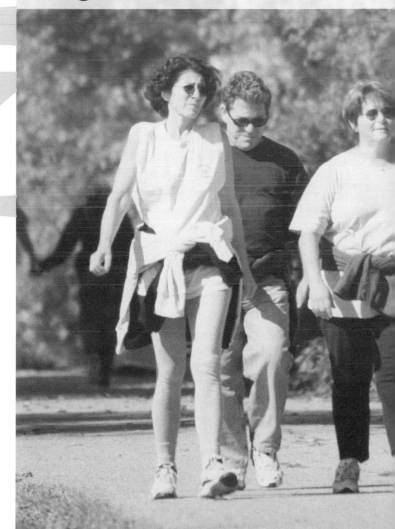

NINE

Using the Stages Model in Group Counseling Programs

Many people find that it is hard to solve physical-activity-related problems on their own. A group physical activity program can offer these people additional ideas about becoming more active through other group members' experiences and thoughts on the subject. Group physical activity programs provide their members with additional channels of social support through relationships with the group members and the group leader. Group members may choose to get together outside of the regular group time and thus provide each other with more regular support. The group leader can facilitate this by encouraging group members to share their phone numbers and call each other during tough times or for problem solving and support. Finally, group counseling has the benefit of being a cost- and time-effective way for health promoters to help several people at once.

There are many types of groups that can promote physical activity. People engaging in physical activity in the same place, such as a gym or pool, or an instructor leading a group of people in an exercise class can be considered a group program. Other groups are more accurately described as health educational, as they offer information related to physical activity. Still others provide both health education and specific skill-building strategies and behavioral techniques that apply psychological theory to behavior change. One example of a program like this is Project Active, discussed in chapter 6 and also later in this chapter (Dunn, Marcus, Kampert, Garcia, Kohl, & Blair, 1999). Then there are groups that are more psychotherapeutic in nature in that they help clients to explore personal habits, emotions, and relationships that affect physical activity habits and use interactions between group members as a means of raising issues and providing feedback related to physical activity. Whether you create a group that is health educational, behavioral skill building, psychotherapeutic, or a group exercise class depends on the setting, your professional training, your style as a group leader, and the needs of your clients. Our purpose in this chapter is to discuss strategies for incorporating the stages of motivational readiness model in group programs that teach members behavioral skills that allow them to be more active outside of group sessions and to incorporate physical activity into their daily lives.

Leading a Stage-Based Group

Group programs are likely to be influenced by the group members' stage of motivational readiness for change and by your role and teaching style as a group leader (Rinne & Toropainen, 1998). You are the group leader presumably because you possess information and expertise that your clients do not. Therefore, one of your roles is to provide information that you have gained in your professional training. You are likely to adopt the role of *teacher* and use a didactic leadership style more often for clients who are in the earlier stages of motivational readiness (stage 1, not thinking about change, and stage 2, thinking about change). For clients in stage 2, thinking about change, and stage 3, doing some physical activity, you may find yourself being a *motivator* who encourages them to try out new skills. For clients in stages 3 (doing some activity) and 4 (doing enough activity), you can also be less didactic and serve more as a *facilitator* who encourages group members to share ideas, experiences, and support. For clients in the later stages 4 and 5 (doing enough physical activity and making physical activity a habit, respectively), you will probably find that you need to give even less information but rather serve as an *analyzer* who helps your clients identify potential pitfalls and as a *consultant* who offers suggestions for avoiding them or handling them better. As the group leader, your flexible use of roles and instructional styles can help you deal with the group as a whole despite the different stages of change of individual group members (Rinne & Toropainen, 1998). Table 9.1 describes teaching styles and instructor roles suited to each of the stages of motivational readiness.

Table 9.1   Group Leader's Role and Teaching Style

Stage	Leader's role	Teaching style	Sample input
1: Not thinking about change	Teacher	Share information	"Let me share with you some ways that physical activity might benefit you, some of which you may not have thought about."
2: Thinking about change	Teacher	Share information	"Research studies have shown that taking a 10-minute walk has important health benefits."
	Motivator	Provide encouragement, increase confidence	"To start out, just do what you feel comfortable with, such as a 5- or 10-minute walk. You sound ready to move on to this step."

(continued)

Table 9.1 *(continued)*

Stage	Leader's role	Teaching style	Sample input
3: Doing some activity	Teacher	Share information	"One of the most helpful ways of making activity a part of your life is to monitor your progress and to give yourself rewards. Let me share with you some ways you might go about doing this."
	Motivator	Provide encouragement	"You are making great progress. You should reward yourself for all your hard work."
	Facilitator	Promote group process (e.g., idea sharing and support among group members)	"What strategies have others tried for fitting in physical activity during a hectic day?"
4: Doing enough activity	Facilitator	Promote group process	"Let's all brainstorm some ideas for what to tell yourself when you don't feel motivated."
	Analyzer	Help identify potential pitfalls	"I've noticed that you really enjoy outdoor activities. Any thoughts on what you are going to do this fall when the weather gets colder?"
	Consultant	Suggest strategies for preventing relapse (e.g., avoiding pitfalls, better handling of pitfalls)	"It sounds like activity is one of the first things to go when you have a lot on your plate. One thing others have found helpful is to try being active first thing in the morning rather than waiting until after work when they are tired and need to take care of their families. Let's talk about how you might do this."
5: Making activity a habit	Motivator	Provide encouragement	"You are active at the level recommended by health experts and have been able to keep it up. Even though you

Stage	Leader's role	Teaching style	Sample input
			may not be an athlete or a 'hard-core' exerciser, I hope you think of yourself as an active person."
	Facilitator	Promote group process	"Why don't we go around the room and say what strategies have been most helpful for keeping active over the long term."
	Analyzer	Help identify potential pitfalls	"It seems that many of you have found an activity or two that you really enjoy. This is great, but one thing we worry about is people's becoming bored with the same routine over time. Let's discuss ways to prevent this."
	Consultant	Suggest strategies for preventing relapse	"Have you thought about what you would do if you were to stop being active for a while? This is bound to happen, and it's important to have a backup plan to keep this from making you stop being active altogether."

Setting Up a Stage-Based Group

There are no hard and fast rules about the number of people you should have in a group or the number of sessions you should hold. Groups with fewer members offer more opportunity for participation and instructor attention. Larger groups, on the other hand, are more cost- and time-effective. Both issues are important to keep in mind when deciding the size of a group. Our general guideline is to have a maximum of 15 people if there is to be individual participation. Five people is probably the minimum useful number for idea sharing and discussions among the participants. That way, if a person or two are unable to attend a given session, there will still be enough members present to exchange thoughts and ideas.

As for the duration of the group, Rinne and Toropainen (1998) have suggested that two to three group sessions are not likely to have much impact, while several months of group sessions may become boring. Ten to 12 weekly group sessions are appropriate for group treatment. If the group expresses an interest in continuing to meet, consider having a break at the end of 12 weeks or so and then scheduling a follow-up group in one month so that group members can share their experiences with continuing their activity plans on their own (Rinne & Toropainen, 1998).

If you will be leading a larger group, consider having a colleague serve as a co-leader. It is always nice to have more than one professional perspective and to share the work of preparing for group, facilitating group discussion, and writing chart notes afterward if your setting requires you to do so. If group members are in various stages of motivational readiness and you decide to break them up into smaller groups based on stage, each of the co-leaders can take responsibility for facilitating a subgroup.

Consider whether or not you will call participants who do not show up for a group session or two. Giving "no-shows" a quick call lets them know that you missed their presence in the group. It also gives you a chance to learn whether something about the group made them decide not to attend or whether personal circumstances kept them from coming. Sometimes people drop out because they feel they are not making progress. A quick phone call to these individuals gives you an opportunity to reiterate that people's stages of readiness to make a personal behavior change vary and that attending group sessions should be considered progress in itself. You could also encourage the client to consider one or two individual sessions, if available, to get him back on track before or in addition to his rejoining the group. Whatever your policy on missed sessions, it is a good idea to tell your group what it is at the outset so that they know what to expect.

Defining Individual Goals

As a group instructor, you will be trying to work on the goals of each individual within the group, which can be challenging if the members of your group are at different stages in the change continuum. For instance, one member may have the personal goal of being active at least five days a week for 30 to 45 minutes at a time. Another member might be satisfied if she maintains three days of activity on a steady basis. While for a third group member, trying one 10-minute brisk walk at some point during the course of the group will be a significant achievement. One way to handle individual goal-setting in a group that has members in various stages of motivational readiness is to encourage members in stages 1 and 2 to set mainly process-oriented goals while members in stages 3, 4, and 5 can be encouraged to set both process-oriented and physical activity behavior goals. By process goals, we are referring to behaviors other than actual physical activity behavior that can help a person move along the stage continuum, such as reading about benefits of physical activity, asking someone to be a walking partner, or finding a location to try a different type of physical activity (e.g., a large, empty parking lot to try inline skating for the first time, parks with good hiking trails). These process goals often make good "homework" assignments for group members between formal group sessions.

Physical activity goals are goals related to frequency, duration, intensity, and type of actual physical activity behaviors (e.g., taking three 15-minute brisk walks during a given week, maintaining 150 minutes of moderate-intensity physical activity for the next two months). Too often individuals and exercise promoters focus mainly on the physical activity behavior goals and place much less (or no) emphasis on process goals, thus individuals in the earlier stages drop out because they are not ready to set a physical activity goal. You also will want to help group members to set both short- and long-term goals related to their physical activity behavior. Perhaps you might choose to define short-term goals as those that can be accomplished in the week between group sessions while long-term goals are those that might be accomplished by the end of the group program. Walking the distance to a predetermined destination (e.g., across the state), achieving a fitness level that will allow an individual to participate in a community walk, and achieving enough reward points to cash in for a weekend away are examples of long-term goals.

Regardless of the type of goal, encourage each group member to set goals that are both *realistic* and *evaluative*. By "realistic" we mean that goals should be something that are challenging for clients yet something that they are likely to achieve and thus enhance their confidence in their ability to be active. By "evaluative" we mean goals should be articulated in such a way that the client and others can observe whether the outcome has been achieved. It is difficult to determine if a goal of "becoming healthier" has been achieved, but one can determine if one is able to walk further or if one's cholesterol level has dropped from 220 to 200. Working on goal-setting in a group setting is a great way to teach this important skill. Group members can learn from each other how to articulate an activity goal in such a way that it can be observed and measured, and they can get ideas for their own goals as they listen to others.

Setting goals also provides a format that you can use to structure a standard group session. The following is a suggested format that you can use for each group session:

- Assess how group members did with their individual short-term goals over the past week and assess their progress toward their long-term goal/s.
- Present the topic for the current group session.
- Evaluate whether group members obtained the information they needed or hoped to receive, and if you, as the group leader, covered all the information you had intended to convey for that session.
- Have each member set a short-term physical activity and/or behavioral skill goal for the upcoming week.

To give you an even better idea of how a stage-based physical activity group might work, let us discuss a program that provided stage-based behavioral skills training in a group format. We also provide a sample of the curriculum used in Project Active (table 9.2).

A Sample Stage-Based Curriculum From Project Active

Project Active (Dunn, Garcia, Marcus, Kampert, Kohl, & Blair, 1998; Dunn, Marcus, Kampert, Garcia, Kohl, & Blair, 1997) was a study that compared a traditional, structured, gymnasium-based exercise program with a lifestyle program that emphasized the newer physical activity recommendation to accumulate moderate-intensity activities on most days of the week (NIH, 1996; Pate et al., 1995; USDHHS, 1996). Both programs had a 6-month intensive intervention phase and an 18-month follow-up intervention phase (Dunn et al., 1999). For the first six months, the

Table 9.2 Lifestyle Curriculum and Targeted Behavioral and Cognitive Strategies

Week	Session title and group activity	Behavioral and cognitive processes
1	Getting to Know You—Monitoring sedentary pursuits, substituting active alternatives	Increasing knowledge, substituting alternatives
2	Understanding Barriers—Listing personal barriers and benefits, fitting short bouts of activity into daily life	Comprehending benefits, increasing healthy opportunities
3	Learning More—Setting goals, assessment of enjoyable physical activities, demonstration of energy intensity	Increasing knowledge
4	Enlisting Aid—Identification of social support sources and types of support	Enlisting social support, committing yourself
5	Getting Confidence—Reflection on overcoming barriers, problem solving to overcome obstacles	Increasing self-efficacy
6	Scavenging for Physical Activity—Examining alternative, nontraditional ways to be physically active	Increasing healthy opportunities, substituting alternatives
7	Rewarding Yourself—Choosing appropriate rewards for reaching short- and long-term goals	Rewarding yourself, committing yourself
8	Time Management Prioritizing daily activities to fit in physical activity	Decision making, increasing healthy opportunities
9	Scouting Physical Activity in Your Community—Using maps and resource guides to find new activities	Increasing healthy opportunities, enlisting social support
10	Reviewing Goals–Using a step counter to monitor activity and set goals	Reminding yourself
11	Physical Activity Fair—Discussion and demonstration of favorite physical activities	Committing yourself, increasing self-efficacy
12	Cognitive Restructuring and Relapse Prevention—Learning how to change all-or-none thinking, planning for relapses	Substituting alternatives, comprehending benefits

lifestyle program was delivered as a group program in which participants met with group facilitators for one hour, one night a week for the first four months and then every other week for two more months. Meeting topics were designed to revolve around cognitive and behavioral skill building, developing self-efficacy for physical activity, and solving problems and focusing on individual issues by both group members and facilitators. The goal was to help individuals learn skills to enable them to integrate activities of at least moderate intensity into their daily life. As self-efficacy and use of the cognitive and behavioral skills increased, the program tapered to fewer (monthly and then bimonthly) group meetings throughout the remainder of the two-year program.

The lifestyle approach used the stages of motivational readiness for change (Prochaska & DiClemente, 1983) and social cognitive theory (Bandura, 1986) as the theoretical framework for shaping physical activity behavior in a manner that takes into account each individual's motivational readiness for change. At the outset of this program, individuals were assessed and told their stage of motivational readiness (e.g., stage 2, thinking about change). Each month for the next six months, their motivational readiness for physical activity was assessed, and they were given a stage-matched physical activity manual (the content of these manuals is discussed in chapter 6). These manuals have been shown to be effective at enhancing physical activity behavior (Marcus, Banspach, Lefebvre, Rossi, Carleton, & Abrams, 1992; Marcus, Bock, Pinto, Forsyth, Roberts, & Traficante, 1998; Marcus, Emmons, et al., 1998). They also were informed that their program goal was to accumulate at least 30 minutes of moderate-intensity activity on most days of the week (Pate et al., 1995; USDHHS, 1996). Participants were instructed to tell program staff their individual goals for becoming more physically active. All of these were interwoven into group discussions and activities.

Incorporated in the lifestyle group meeting curriculum were the 10 processes of change, self-efficacy, and decision-making for physical activity (see chapters 2, 3, and 4), which are part of the stages of motivational readiness for change model (Prochaska & DiClemente, 1983) and social cognitive theory (Bandura, 1986) that can be applied to physical activity adoption and maintenance. These ideas were the basis of the strategies for building self-efficacy and cognitive and behavioral skills. For example, increasing knowledge is one of the five cognitive processes of change and can include increasing knowledge about the importance of physical activity and increasing knowledge about one's own sedentary habits. During one of the first lifestyle group meetings, participants were asked to complete a one-week log of the time they spent sitting. At the next session, they shared their results with the group, and each person developed a plan within the context of their stage of motivational readiness and life circumstance to decrease the amount of time spent sitting. Samples of activities from the six-month curriculum and the corresponding psychological processes are shown in table 9.2. The full curriculum is available in the book *Active Living Every Day* (Blair, Dunn, Marcus, Carpenter, & Jaret, 2001).

Assessing Whether You Met Your Objective for a Session

To determine whether you, as the group leader, achieved your objective for a session or topic, you can use group discussion and feedback. Another means of assessment is to choose some written questions that go over group content. For instance, if the topic of the group session was self-efficacy, you might want to have the group complete the questionnaire found in chapter 5 at the beginning of the group so that group members can identify areas in which they are more or less confident. Then after spending the group session discussing ways to stay active in challenging situations such as vacations and bad weather, you might have the group again answer the questions to see if there have been any improvements in self-efficacy. If there is no standardized measure available for the topic you covered, you can write out a few questions on the content that you hope to cover and the group can see how well they learned the information. You do not necessarily have to collect their responses, but rather have this exercise be a way for each group member to collect information about himself. If you do decide to collect their answers, you may opt to keep the identity of each respondent anonymous so that the information you collect is more honest. Alternatively, you could have group members put their names on the questionnaires and then write out specific feedback or ways they might want to try to increase confidence in the areas in which they are struggling. You may also want to encourage each group member to keep a diary in between group sessions as a way to track progress and to jot down issues as they arise for discussion at the next group. Some examples of useful content to include in a diary are provided in chapter 7.

Suggestions for Stage-Specific Group Activities

The following provides some topics and activities that can be incorporated into your own group curriculum. You can select among the different options based on the stage/s of motivational readiness of your group members. If your group consists mainly of individuals who are in the same or similar stages of change, you might use the strategies described under the appropriate stage. If you find that your group has members in both the earliest stages (e.g., 1 or 2) and the later stages (e.g., 4 or 5), you might find it easier to break up the group into smaller subgroups to adequately address the needs of each of your members. We would also encourage you to come up with your own ideas for group activities based on your setting and the needs of your clients.

STAGE 1

Not Thinking About Change

You may find that some of the individuals in this earliest stage are enrolled in your group but are not interested in considering physical activity at the present time. Perhaps they joined to please someone else such as a physician or family member. Or, maybe they initially joined the group because they were in stages 2 or 3 but then regressed to this stage sometime during the course of the group. We suggest that you let them know they can still attend the group meetings even if they are not interested in starting activity right now, because they may get some ideas that will be helpful if they should want to be active later on. You might try some of the following strategies to get them to think about trying physical activity again or perhaps for the first time.

What might you do to keep these individuals involved in your group?

- Determine their willingness to participate in discussions or do other behavioral assignments such as looking up benefits of physical activity.
- Lead a discussion about how a person's sedentary behavior might affect those around them.
- Discuss another relevant health behavior (e.g., smoking cessation, healthy eating) and incorporate the relationship of physical activity with this behavior.
- Discuss past attempts at becoming physically active. Is this related to why someone is not interested in change now?
- Ask if you can check in with them every month or so to see where they are with physical activity.
- Foster social support from other group members for someone who is still attending the group meetings even though she is not thinking about becoming physically active now.

What are the barriers?

- Administer the PAR-Q and address health events as a reason for not considering physical activity.
- Lead a group discussion on true barriers versus excuses.
- Consider addressing body image. Listen for any clues, which suggest that some members are resistant to becoming physically active because they are embarrassed by how they would look engaged in physical activity.

(continued)

(continued)

What information might these group members need to consider physical activity?

- Present new recommended levels of physical activity and the benefits that can be gained through accumulated moderate-intensity physical activities.

- Describe a list of lifestyle activities that can help a person achieve health benefits if performed at a moderate intensity. Notions of "no pain, no gain" may be leading some to remain at this stage.

- Invite a guest speaker to give a presentation on the benefits of physical activity.

What goals might help these individuals move toward considering change?

- Reinforce the idea that achieving other behavioral or cognitive goals, even if they do not include actual physical activity, are productive and worthwhile.

- Have these group members think about a behavior, other than physical activity, which they were successful at changing, and generate a list of strategies that were helpful in these past attempts. You can write them on a blackboard or a big sheet of paper to help others get ideas for physical activity behavior change.

- Have group members generate common negative thoughts concerning physical activity and identify an alternative positive thought they could use to replace it.

STAGE 2

Thinking About Change

Group members in this stage are thinking about becoming more active and will probably find support from other group members helpful in their efforts to move toward actually trying this new behavior. Ideas from other group members who are participating in physical activity can help members in stage 2 to carefully plan their initial attempts at physical activity so that the experience is pleasant enough to try it again. Here are some ideas for helping group members who are thinking about change.

What information might help these group members to consider trying some physical activity?

- Present new physical activity recommendations and the benefits that can be gained through accumulated moderate-intensity physical activities.
- Describe a list of lifestyle activities that can help a person achieve health benefits if performed at a moderate intensity. Notions of "no pain, no gain" may be preventing some from becoming physically active.
- Present different types of social support (described in chapter 4). Have each individual identify areas in which social support would be helpful to her in getting started.
- Invite a guest speaker to give a presentation on the benefits of physical activity.
- Lead a discussion about how a person's sedentary behavior might affect those around them.
- Discuss another relevant health behavior (e.g., smoking cessation, healthy eating) and incorporate the relationship of physical activity with this behavior.

What are the barriers?

- Use the IDEA approach described in chapter 8 to teach group members how to overcome perceived barriers. Have group members practice this problem-solving approach with each other or on their own.
- Consider addressing body image during one of the groups. Listen for any clues, which suggest that some members have put off becoming physically active because they are embarrassed by how they would look engaged in physical activity.
- Discuss past attempts at becoming physically active. Is this related to why some group members are not physically active now or have low confidence?

(continued)

(continued)

- Lead a group discussion on true barriers versus excuses for not trying physical activity.
- Lead a group discussion on priority setting and where beginning physical activity fits in their list of priorities.

What kinds of activities might help with getting started?

- Set up teams among group members to investigate different aspects of physical activity (e.g., benefits of cardiovascular activities, benefits of weight training, mental health benefits, local places to go swing dancing).
- Through group discussion, develop strategies for obtaining social support and rewarding others who provide social support.
- Have group members generate common negative thoughts concerning physical activity. Have each group member identify an alternative positive thought they could use to replace it. For this activity, it is important that each person identify an alternative statement that will work for him.
- Discuss activities that members in this stage might like to try or find enjoyable. Encourage group members to plan when, where, and with whom they might try some of these activities.
- Think of ways in which some light activities can be stepped up a notch into moderate-intensity activities.
- Post the commit dates for trying a physical activity on a bulletin board or on a handout.

What goals might help these individuals move toward considering change?

- Ask group members to talk to someone they know who was successful at becoming physically active and get their advice. Have them share this advice with other group members at the next meeting.
- Have each group member complete a personal time study in which she monitors time spent sitting and time spent engaging in some physical activity during two typical weekdays and a typical weekend day. Spend part of the next group meeting brainstorming ideas for decreasing sedentary time and increasing time spent in physical activity.
- Ask group members to look up information about physical activity and its benefits or discover interesting Web sites about physical activity as a homework assignment. Have the group members take turns reporting their findings at their next meeting.
- Plan a 10-minute walk either during group time or for individuals to try on their own during the next week.

STAGE 3

Doing Some Physical Activity

Participants in this stage are doing some physical activity but not enough. Group discussion that provides these individuals with additional ideas and strategies for increasing their activity level will be helpful for these individuals, as will support from other group members. Be sure to encourage goal setting for both behavioral skills and actual physical activity behaviors. Here are some ideas for group members in this stage.

What are the remaining barriers?

- Choose an obstacle that is interfering with physical activity for one or several of the group members. Demonstrate how to use the IDEA approach described in chapter 8 to develop potential solutions for overcoming this barrier. Practice with other obstacles.
- Give a presentation on time management.
- Lead a group discussion on true barriers versus excuses for not increasing one's physical activity.

What information might help to increase physical activity?

- Discuss how to make small environmental changes (e.g., move home exercise equipment from a seldom used spare bedroom to the room where the TV is located) that can help to promote physical activity.
- Teach group members different strategies for incorporating short bouts of physical activity into their daily lives.
- Demonstrate energy intensity.
- Work with group members on setting appropriate goals for gradually increasing their physical activity.
- Present different types of social support (described in chapter 4). Have each individual identify areas in which social support would be helpful to him in becoming more active. Through group discussion, develop strategies for obtaining social support and rewarding others who provide social support.
- Generate a list of possible rewards for achieving personal goals. Also describe how one might use a point system to reward progress over time.
- Invite a guest speaker to give a presentation on the benefits of increasing physical activity.
- Describe ways in which some light activities can be stepped up a notch into moderate-intensity activities.

(continued)

(continued)

What kind of activities might help increase physical activity?

- Have group members generate common negative thoughts concerning physical activity. Have each group member identify an alternative positive self-statement they could use to replace it.

- Spend group time completing the Processes-of-Change Questionnaire found on page 61. Spend some additional time having group members identify additional change strategies they might wish to try, and get feedback from others on how these strategies might be implemented.

- Have group members brainstorm different ways they might remind themselves to be more active.

- Lead a group discussion on priority setting and where increasing physical activity fits in their list of priorities.

What goals might help these individuals move toward increasing physical activity participation?

- Ask group members to talk to someone they know who was successful at becoming regularly active and get their advice. Have them share this advice with other group members at the next meeting.

- Have each group member complete a personal time study in which she monitors time spent sitting and time spent engaging in some physical activity during two typical weekdays and one typical weekend day. Spend the next group meeting brainstorming ideas for decreasing sedentary time and increasing time spent in physical activity.

- Encourage group members to try a new type of physical activity. You might have some group members give a short presentation on the activities they like to do.

- Encourage short-term physical activity goals that are realistic and manageable. For example, individuals in stage 3 might consider increasing their current duration of physical activity per day by 5 or 10 minutes or their frequency of physical activity by one day.

STAGE 4

Doing Enough Physical Activity

Even though these group members are physically active at the recommended level, their challenge will be to maintain physical activity over time. They will still benefit from information you present to them and from setting both behavioral and physical activity goals. Here are some suggestions for helping regularly active group members keep it up.

What information might help with sticking with physical activity until it is a habit?

- Encourage group members to share ideas on alternative activities to help prevent boredom.
- Lead a discussion concerning how others can unintentionally (or intentionally) try to sabotage one's best efforts to stay active. How have others overcome this issue? Discuss how group members have encouraged others to be appropriately supportive.
- Invite a guest lecturer to talk about or demonstrate a new type of activity such as tai chi, yoga, or kick boxing.
- Pass out information on local hiking or biking trails.
- Discuss different ways to monitor activity such as activity logs, perceived exertion, or heart rate (see chapter 7).
- Present on the importance of rewarding oneself for accomplishing personal goals.
- Present on common obstacles that arise and get even the most dedicated exercisers off track (see chapter 7).
- Suggest the use of a step counter to monitor activity and set goals. Bring one in and demonstrate how to set, wear, and read it. Present different ways to use the step counter for setting goals and monitoring progress.
- Invite a guest speaker to give a presentation on the benefits of regular physical activity.
- Teach group members different strategies for incorporating short bouts of physical activity into their daily life.

What kinds of goals might help maintain physical activity?

- Try a new activity as a group (e.g., ice skating at a nearby rink).
- Encourage group members to identify a role model that helps to motivate them.
- Have group members generate a personal list of rewards.

(continued)

(continued)

- Ask group members to generate a list of what they have given up to become physically active or what they still find unpleasant about physical activity. Discuss alternative ways to address these issues.
- Work on appropriate goal setting to maintain motivation over the long-term.
- Go around the room and have individuals say what types of benefits they feel they have already achieved. What benefits are they still working toward?
- Problem-solve around any remaining obstacles some group members may still be experiencing.
- Have group members brainstorm some different ways they might post reminders in their environment that encourage them to praise themselves for their success.

STAGE 5

Making Physical Activity a Habit

Participants in this stage are quite knowledgeable about physical activity. However, group meetings can still be a valuable source of support and a forum for getting additional ideas. Having "booster" sessions once a month or so may remind stage 5 individuals to review what has helped them remain active, encourage them to think of new ways to keep activity enjoyable, and formulate a plan for any future setbacks. Here are some ideas for group activities relevant to individuals who have managed to keep active over time.

What kind of group activities might foster continued physical activity maintenance?

- Encourage group members to share ideas on alternative activities to help prevent boredom.
- Invite a guest lecturer to talk about or demonstrate a new type of activity such as spinning, cross-country skiing, or in-line skating.
- Try a new activity as a group (e.g., rock climbing at an indoor facility).
- Pass out information on local hiking or biking trails.
- Discuss different ways to monitor activity (see chapter 7).
- Present on the importance of continuing to reward oneself for achieving personal goals. Have group members generate a personal list of rewards. Be sure to describe how one might use a point system to reward progress over time.
- Work on appropriate goal setting to maintain motivation over the long term.
- Spend time identifying possible setbacks and developing plans to prepare for and overcome them.
- Have participants try to think of alternative, non-traditional ways to be active.
- Encourage these individuals to become a physical activity mentor to someone whom they know is less active.
- Present on how members can change all-or-none thinking should they find themselves getting off track.
- Ask these group members to generate a list of what they have given up to remain physically active or what they still find unpleasant about physical activity. Discuss alternative ways to address these issues.

CONCLUSION

Although tailoring a client's program based on his stage of motivational readiness seems like an individual approach for promoting physical activity, it can be successfully used in a group setting, as this chapter describes. Your role as the group leader varies, depending on the stage of motivational readiness of your group members. The goals that you set for your group and the goals of each individual in the group also vary according to stage of motivational readiness. You can build the curriculum of your group program around the stages of change and the processes of change, as was done in Project Active. Leading a physical activity group program can be a fun and effective way of sharing ideas and building support for your clients in their efforts to be more physically active.

References

Bandura, A. (1986). *Social foundations of thought and action: A social cognitive theory.* Englewood Cliffs, NJ: Prentice Hall.

Blair, S.N., Dunn, A.L., Marcus, B.H., Carpenter, R.A., & Jaret, P. (2001). *Active living every day.* Champaign, IL: Human Kinetics.

Dunn, A.L., Garcia, M.E., Marcus, B.H., Kampert, J.B., Kohl, H.W., & Blair, S.N. (1998). Six-month physical activity and fitness changes in Project Active, a randomized trial. *Medicine and Science in Sports and Exercise, 30,* 1076–1083.

Dunn, A.L., Marcus, B.H., Kampert, J.B., Garcia, M.E., Kohl, H.W., III, & Blair, S.N. (1997). Reduction in cardiovascular disease risk factors: 6-month results from Project Active. *Preventive Medicine, 26,* 883–892.

Dunn, A.L., Marcus, B.H., Kampert, J.B., Garcia, M.E., Kohl, H.W., III, & Blair, S.N. (1999). Project Active: A 24-month randomized trial to compare lifestyle and structured physical activity interventions. *Journal of the American Medical Association, 281,* 327–334.

Marcus, B.H., Banspach, S.W., Lefebvre, R.C., Rossi, J.S., Carleton, R.A., & Abrams D.B. (1992). Using the stages of change model to increase the adoption of physical activity among community participants. *American Journal of Health Promotion, 6,* 424–429.

Marcus, B.H., Bock, B.C., Pinto, B.M., Forsyth, L.H., Roberts, M., & Traficante, R. (1998). Efficacy of individualized, motivationally tailored physical activity intervention. *Annals of Behavioral Medicine, 20,* 174–180.

Marcus, B.H., Emmons, K.M., Simkin-Silverman, L.R., Linnan, L.A., Taylor, E.R., Bock, B.C., et al. (1998). Evaluation of stage-matched versus standard self-help physical activity interventions at the workplace. *American Journal of Health Promotion, 12,* 246–253.

NIH Consensus Development Panel on Physical Activity and Cardiovascular Health. (1996). NIH Consensus Conference: Physical activity and cardiovascular health. *Journal of the American Medical Association, 276,* 241–246.

Pate, R.R., Pratt, M., Blair, S.N., Haskell, W.L., Macera, C.A., Bouchard, C., et al. (1995). Physical activity and public health: A recommendation from the Centers for Disease Control and Prevention and the American College of Sports Medicine. *Journal of the American Medical Association, 273,* 402–407.

Prochaska, J.O., & DiClemente, C.C. (1983). The stages and processes of self-change in smoking: Towards an integrative model of change. *Journal of Consulting and Clinical Psychology, 51,* 390–395.

Rinne, M., & Toropainen, E. (1998). How to lead a group: Practical principles and experiences of conducting a promotional group in health-related physical activity. *Patient Education and Counseling, 33,* S69–S76.

U.S. Department of Health and Human Services. (1996). *Physical activity and health: A report of the Surgeon General.* Atlanta, GA: Centers for Disease Control and Prevention, National Center for Chronic Disease Prevention and Health Promotion.

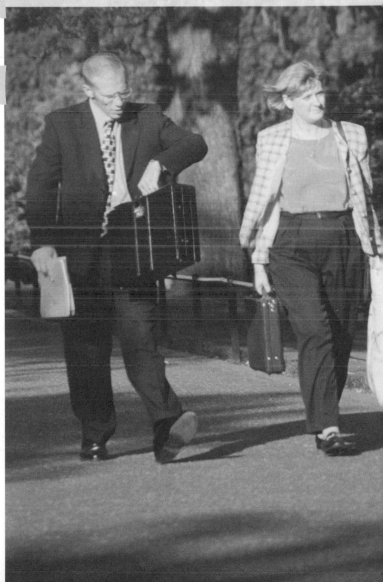

TEN

Using the Stages Model in Work-Site Programs

Between 110 and 115 million Americans go to work each day, and this number is estimated to increase to between 141 and 153 million people by the year 2010 (USDHHS, 1993). Therefore, physical activity programs for workplaces offer great opportunities for helping a lot of sedentary people become more active. However, many people probably feel that the hours they spend at work interfere with the time they have available for physical activity. This does not have to be the case.

The work setting can be an ideal place for disseminating physical-activity-related information. Office settings typically have communication channels in place, such as voice mail, the company computer network, newsletters, and mail boxes, that can be useful for providing factual information or spreading information about physical activity opportunities. In other workplaces, such as factories and retail settings, where employees may not have access to computer networks or voice mail, other channels such as paycheck stuffers and bulletin boards can be used to get the word out about physical activity programs you are offering.

Also, work environments can be arranged to provide opportunities for actual physical activity. Reminders to use the stairwell instead of the elevator can be posted, walking routes both inside the building and outside on the grounds can be marked and measured, and exercise equipment and facilities can even be provided. Furthermore, the hours that employees spend at work actually can provide hidden opportunities for activity so that they can go home having already accumulated 30 minutes. Using coffee breaks to take quick 5- or 10-minute walks, holding one-on-one meetings while walking, and using the stairs instead of the elevator are examples of how this can be done. Finally, many work sites offer a built-in social support network that you can use to spread your message and support employees in their efforts to be more active.

However, work-site programs traditionally recruit only about 20 percent of employees (Wanzel, 1994). This figure drops to only 10 percent of the employee population after taking into account typical dropout rates for such programs. Furthermore, the employees who are attracted to work-site programs tend to be the people who are already active to some degree (Sharratt & Cox, 1988; Shephard, 1992). However, work-site programs based on the stages of motivational readiness model take a more proactive stance by attempting to reach even those who are not interested in making behavior change in the foreseeable future. Work-site programs that foster a more positive attitude toward physical activity and create a social norm that supports good health and positive health habits may move the most unmotivated individuals closer to adopting some physical activity or at least thinking about becoming more active in the near future (USDHHS et al., 1999). These employees may later decide to participate in activity either at home or at a different facility within their community. This chapter discusses general issues regarding the stage-matched approach for work-site programs and specific strategies that can be implemented in stage-matched workplace interventions.

Building Support for Your Program

Before you begin developing and implementing your work-site program, you are obviously going to need to consider the employer's commitment to your efforts. For example, if you want employees to participate in assessments of motivational readiness while at work, then managerial support for using work time for this purpose is clearly necessary. Selling your program as a benefit to the employer through increasing the mental and physical well-being of the staff is well worth your time and effort. In a work-site program we recently implemented simultaneously in a U.S. work site and an Australian work site, recruitment and retention of employees was dramatically better in the Australian work site. The primary reason was that the Australian CEO supported the program and told employees that he thought it was a good use of their time to read through the materials and think about becoming more active. This does not mean that you cannot accomplish important goals without support from high-level management. You just may need more modest goals, and you need to make it clear to employees that you are delivering a home-based program through their workplace.

Assessing Motivational Readiness

Because movement among the stages of motivational readiness is a dynamic process, to target your program you need a means of assessing each employee's stage of motivational readiness that is quick and easy for both the employee and the program administrators. The paper-and-pencil measure in chapter 2 can be answered quickly, and scoring it takes little time. It is also easy to train someone to do the scoring. However, in a pilot work-site project we conducted, we found that written assessments were often lost in piles of paper on employees' desks or left at home. Also, employees became less interested in the program in the few days that it took us to receive their questionnaires by interoffice mail and then send out stage-matched materials. Asking the five stage-determining questions by phone proved to be worth the extra effort in our program. When we determined an employee's stage of readiness for change over the phone, we were able to send out the stage-matched materials to arrive the very next day. Although this direct contact required extra time on our part and was more troublesome, we felt that it helped to engage employees in the program. In work settings where employees do not have private access to a telephone, a short questionnaire that can be dropped into a convenience box on site is another way to quickly do stage assessment and thus minimize the delay for delivering stage-targeted materials.

If some component of your program requires registration, such as a seminar or skills-building class, consider putting the stage-assessing questions from chapter 2 on the registration form so that you can better match the message delivered during the event. If your program does not require registration, consider having employees complete the stage-assessing questions as a way of entering a prize drawing (Glaros, 1997). Because entering the drawing does not necessarily commit the employee to any part of the physical activity program, this suggestion is a good way to get a fairly accurate idea of where employees lie on the stages-of-change continuum.

Because people's stage of readiness to change fluctuates, you should assess employees' stages at several points in the program, depending on its length. Some programs have conducted stage assessments at the beginning, at one month, and at three months (Marcus et al., 1998); however, there is no hard and fast rule for how often stage assessment should be done. How frequently you assess participants' behavior and physical activity intentions and what you use to assess their behavior depends on your program goals and ultimately the type of change you need to be able to demonstrate in order to continue receiving funding or to attract new funding for your program.

Choosing Your Target Audience

When designing your work-site program, one of your first decisions will be if you will take a reactive stance (i.e., potential participants come to you) or a proactive stance (i.e., you reach out to potential participants and offer your services) to participant recruitment. If you decide to start with reactive recruitment strategies, you will need to have ideas for helping individuals at different stages of motivational readiness. However, if you proactively recruit participants, you can decide which stage you want your program to target and how you will reach those individuals. For example, you may want your first program to focus on those in stage 3, who do some physical activity each week. Your job is to help them become regular exercisers. These individuals are an easy first target for your program because they are likely to be quite receptive to physical activity messages and events, and they have some ideas about how to get started. To reach them, you could conduct and publicize a fun event, such as an "exercise journey" in which you pick a destination, such as New Orleans during Mardi Gras season; track the time or miles it would take to walk, jog, or swim there; and reward individuals when they accomplish the journey (Glaros, 1997). Such an event promotes the idea that physical activity is important and fun and also encourages your target group members to monitor their progress and reward themselves for reaching a goal. If this event is successful, you can plan how to reach employees at other stages.

Although already active, employees in stage 4, doing enough physical activity, and stage 5, making it a habit, are often the individuals most interested in physical activity programs offered at work. Special events such as a fun run, fitness assessment, or reward for physical activity participation can keep them motivated by making their physical activity fun and different from their ordinary routine. Employees in these stages also are likely to be interested in tips for maintaining their activity during difficult times, such as bad weather or illness, and in information about unfamiliar exercise benefits, such as improved immune functioning. These tips and information can be provided in a short monthly newsletter or an e-mail message. That these individuals are already active at the recommended levels does not mean that they have little to gain from physical activity promotion. In fact, helping them vary their activities to prevent boredom and relapse is especially important for physical activity behavior, which is characterized by several starts and stops during a person's lifetime.

Employees in the earliest stages (i.e., stage 1, not thinking about change, and stage 2, thinking about change) are probably the audience that health promoters most want to reach, but their lack of motivational readiness makes them the hardest to involve in work-site physical activity events. Your task is to increase these individuals' awareness of the importance of physical activity, reinforce the notion that *anyone* can be physically active, and get them to think about how their current inactivity might affect them and others who are important to them. For this group, motivationally targeted messages that acknowledge their reluctance to become physically active are paramount. For example, ideas for overcoming common barriers may attract these individuals' attention because they feel that the reasons for being inactive outweigh those for being active. A heading such as "Not Ready to Be Physically Active?" communicates to employees at early stages that the information provided is relevant to them. Messages aimed at individuals in the earlier stages and events for employees in the later stages communicate to all employees that physical activity is important and valued by the employer. This recognition that physical activity is valued by one's employer can be crucial in moving individuals even in the earliest stages toward actually taking part in some physical activity.

Reaching Your Target Audience

A common way to communicate physical activity messages at the workplace is to post them in highly visible places: bulletin boards, the cafeteria, doorways. Sending questions and receiving answers by e-mail is another good option for many work sites. However, individuals who do not have a current interest in becoming more physically active may not pay much attention to these messages or may quickly dismiss them as irrelevant. Therefore, consider other communication routes that employees routinely use: office mail, paycheck stuffers, voice mail, a brief announcement on the company's intranet. Messages from managers, other employees, the human resources department, employee assistance programs, union leaders, and so forth may convince individuals at the early stages of motivational readiness to at least give physical activity another thought (USDHHS et al., 1999). Using several channels of communication also demonstrates to the employees the organization's commitment to physical activity promotion.

Developing Stage-Matched Materials

In addition to written materials that describe the different exercise facilities available, how to start an exercise program (e.g., brochures from the AHA such as "Exercise and Your Heart: A Guide to Physical Activity" and "The Walking Handbook"), and so on, be sure to also have available materials geared toward people not thinking about activity and those thinking about it but not yet ready to start. Such materials might include a handout on the benefits of regular activity or suggestions for how to deal with common barriers that keep people from exercising. In materials such as these, be sure to applaud the employee for taking the important step of picking up the brochure and reading about exercise. It is helpful to acknowledge in the title or the opening text that the reader may not be thinking of starting a physical activity program now but that the information might be useful if the person starts thinking more seriously about becoming physically active in the future. For example, we have used titles such as "What's in It for Me?" and "Do I Need This?" on materials designed for people in stage 1. This helps readers in the early stages to perceive the materials as relevant to them and thereby increases the likelihood that they will actually read the materials. Those in the later stages are looking for different information, such as how to prevent injury, how to add variety to their usual physical activity routine, or suggestions for being active during vacations or business trips. Following are some suggested topics for stage-matched written materials.[1]

Topics for Creating Stage-Appropriate Materials

Stage 1: Not thinking about change

- Health benefits of physical activity
- Overcoming common excuses

Stage 2: Thinking about change

- Increasing lifestyle activity
- Considering benefits and barriers
- Setting short- and long-term goals
- Rewarding yourself

Stage 3: Doing some physical activity

- Goal setting
- Developing a walking program

---

[1]Copies of stage-matched materials that have been developed and tested in work settings can be ordered by calling 401-793-8176 or e-mailing a request to LSExercise@lifespan.org.

- Tips for enjoying physical activity
- Fitting more activity into a busy schedule

Stage 4: Doing enough physical activity

- Overcoming obstacles
- Preventing boredom
- Gaining social support
- Increasing your confidence in staying active

Stage 5: Making physical activity a habit

- Avoiding injury
- Trying new activities
- Planning ahead for difficult situations
- Rewarding yourself

Focusing on Moderate-Intensity Activity

Many individuals still adhere to the old adage "no pain, no gain" when it comes to physical activity. This philosophy is particularly unappealing to those who are not motivated to be more physically active. A worksite program based on the stages of motivational readiness for change should promote activities that do not take much time or effort, consistent with the philosophy that a little activity is better than none at all. Examples of such activities include taking the stairs rather than the elevator once in a while, parking in the farthest parking space for one day, or taking a walking break. Ask managers to provide their employees with opportunities for physical activity to increase the effectiveness of your program.

Some businesses and employers might be reluctant to promote physical activity because they are concerned about liability issues should an employee become injured through physical activity promoted in their workplace. However, asking each employee to consult with a physician first puts up another barrier. You can address this concern by letting the employer know that you advocate moderate-intensity activity. Using the Physical Activity Readiness Questionnaire (PAR-Q; see chapter 8) to identify any potential health concerns can allay employers' concerns about this issue.

Planning Events

Ideas for action-oriented events for the workplace, such as walk-a-thons or using a map of the United States to track miles, are readily available (e.g., Glaros, 1997). However, a stage-matched workplace program also should include events that are more personal and informational in nature, such as walking programs, structured classes, and skill-building programs. An example of an event for employees in early stages of motivational readiness is a barriers assessment in which employees take a minute or two to identify their top few reasons for not becoming physically active (they can use the form in figure 8.4 in chapter 8) and then use problem-solving strategies to overcome these barriers. This activity can be done in either an individual or a group format. Another idea is to have employees identify how they might personally benefit from becoming a little more physically active and perhaps sharing this information with a family member or co-worker. Finding an article or Web site (e.g., **www.americanheart.org**) that pertains to physical activity could be a short-term goal for those in the earlier stages. This might also provide you with useful materials to distribute to other employees. Increasing employees' awareness of your program can be accomplished by kicking off your program with a guest speaker or a gift given to each employee, such as a T-shirt, shoelaces, or a water bottle.

Employees in the early stages of motivational readiness may not be interested in becoming more physically active at present, but they might be interested in related issues, such as managing their weight, quitting smoking, lowering stress, or time management. Addressing these topics can enhance their confidence that they can use their new time management skills to become active or persuade them that a little physical activity can be helpful in their efforts to manage their weight. These topics also are likely to be relevant to people in stages 3, 4, and 5 and may help them increase or maintain their activity. Thus, programs addressing these topics can be a great use of your time and of management's financial resources.

Incentives for Participation

A review of workplace physical activity interventions found that adding incentives for participation in a program helped the program to be even more effective (Dishman, Oldenburg, O'Neal, & Shephard, 1998).

Including several incentives for participation, especially in the beginning, helps make employees committed to the program. Incentives can be financial, such as additional payment or reimbursement for participation. An employer might collaborate with a local exercise facility to offer a one-month membership to the facility for employees who sign up for the program. Prizes such as T-shirts either for participation or for achievement of physical activity goals also have been used. However, it is important to ensure that the goals to be attained are commensurate with the individual employee's baseline motivation level; one employee may hit his goal by reading about physical activity five days that week, while another employee may need to participate in physical activity five days that week to meet her goal. Awards and recognition through trophies, certificates, or announcements in the workplace help create a social norm for physical activity. Listing participants' names in an employee newsletter can also be effective. Release time from work to participate also has been used as an incentive to get employees to participate, although this obviously requires management's support.

Stage-Specific Strategies for Workplace Programs

Once you have evaluated employee interest and managerial support for your work-site physical activity promotion program, funds available, and the means that you are going to use to deliver your program, it is time to put it together. We hope that the following list of stage-specific workplace program strategies will help you generate some ideas for the type of program that will meet the needs of the employees with whom you are working.

STAGE 1

Not Thinking About Change

For sedentary employees who are not thinking about physical activity behavior change, an appropriate objective for your program might be to increase their awareness of the benefits of physical activity and the level of activity necessary to obtain these benefits. Here are some strategies for increasing awareness and encouraging these employees to begin to think about the role physical activity could play in their lives.

What are some ways to promote physical activity awareness?

- Kick off your program with a special event such as a guest speaker, or giving T-shirts to every employee (USDHHS et al., 1999).
- Set up informational displays in prominent places such as the front entrance, reception areas, by the elevator or stairwell, on bulletin boards, at coffee or snack machines, in the restrooms, or by e-mail (USDHHS et al., 1999).
- Offer an incentive to employees who read or find information on physical activity.
- Distribute print materials targeted toward individuals who are presently not thinking about becoming more physically active.
- Host a health fair during lunch that includes fitness testing, blood pressure screenings, or body fat assessments. Relate how these are affected by physical activity.

What information might get employees to consider physical activity?

- Give a presentation to correct common misconceptions (e.g., you have to exercise vigorously to gain health benefits).
- Present new recommended levels of physical activity and the benefits that can be gained through accumulated moderate-intensity physical activities.
- Describe a list of lifestyle activities that can help a person achieve health benefits if performed at a moderate intensity. Notions of "no pain, no gain" may be leading some to remain at this stage.

What are some strategies for making physical activity personally relevant to these employees?

- Conduct a health fair that offers free physical fitness assessments (USDHHS et al., 1999).
- Do a barriers assessment for home or work-site physical activity (depending on the goals of your program) and provide suggestions for overcoming barriers.

(continued)

(continued)

- Have employees identify how they might personally benefit from becoming physically active.
- Help employees see how your message relates to their lives by personalizing the message.
- Hold a workshop or seminar on related topics such as weight loss, time management, stress management, or quitting smoking. Include how physical activity relates to these other areas.
- Find out what the employees in your setting desire most and tailor your activities to those goals (weight loss, health benefits, mental health benefits).

What type of special event is particularly relevant for these employees?

- Hold a "Top Ten Excuses T-Shirt Contest" (Glaros, 1997).

  Ask employees to submit their best excuse for not exercising. Ask for two excuses—one that is a legitimate problem for them and another a humorous excuse. Have the excuses judged by your employee wellness committee or other staff.

  Order your T-shirts with the "Top Ten Excuses" printed on the shirt. Award a free T-shirt to the employees who submitted the selected 10 excuses.

  Offer support, guidance, or suggestions on how to overcome the legitimate excuses for all entrants.

  Use the list of entrants as a targeted mailing list for promotion materials.

STAGE 2
Thinking About Change

For this segment of employees, one of your objectives might be to increase awareness of the benefits of physical activity and its acceptance in the work community. A second objective would be to move these employees closer to actually trying out the behavior. Here are some ideas for achieving these objectives.

What are some ways to promote physical activity awareness?

- Distribute print materials targeted toward individuals who are thinking about becoming more physically active.
- Establish a physical activity library with educational materials on physical activity (USDHHS et al., 1999).
- Take advantage of New Year's resolutions in January, the start of spring, annual employee physicals, or other dates to post information or hold an event (Glaros, 1997).
- Kick off your program with a special event such as a guest speaker, or giving T-shirts to every employee (USDHHS et al., 1999).
- Set up informational displays in prominent places such as the front entrance, reception areas, by the elevator or stairwell, on bulletin boards, at coffee or snack machines, in the restrooms, or by e-mail (USDHHS et al., 1999).
- Offer an incentive to employees who read or find information on physical activity.

What information might get employees to consider physical activity?

- Conduct a health fair that offers free physical fitness assessments (USDHHS et al., 1999).
- Gather and distribute a list of community resources for physical activity (USDHHS et al., 1999).
- Do a barriers assessment for home or work-site physical activity (depending on the goals of your program) and provide suggestions for overcoming barriers.
- Hold a workshop on developing an activity plan (what, where, when, with whom).

What strategies might prompt these employees to try some physical activity?

- Provide employees with the opportunity to take a 10-minute "walk-break" during the workday.

(continued)

(continued)

- Post cues by the elevator to take the stairs instead of the elevator.
- Have employees set up a "start date" during which time they will complete the goal of 10 minutes of physical activity. Follow up to see how the employees did.
- Ask employees to walk to a lunch spot that is a couple of blocks away rather than going to the in-house cafeteria or the place across the street.
- Give the message that "some activity is better than nothing."

What is an example of a special event that would be appropriate for employees in this stage?

- Host an event entitled "Walk a Mall in My Shoes" (Glaros, 1997).

  Plan a walking route that covers an appropriate distance in a mall.

  Select stores at appropriate intervals as checkpoints and record some distinctive feature from their window display like sales prices, featured items, or unique displays. Formulate these facts into a scavenger hunt with a series of questions that participants must answer during the course of the walk.

  Keep in mind that many of the participants will be sedentary, so be conservative with the distance you expect them to travel.

  Encourage participants to walk the route in pairs in the order you have indicated.

  Arrange for gift certificates valid in the mall as incentives.

STAGE 3

Doing Some Physical Activity

Employees in this stage are likely to be receptive to physical activity promotion in the workplace, given that they are doing some activity but not enough to meet national guidelines. Therefore, your program objective for this group is to encourage them to increase the amount of physical activity they do each week, perhaps by getting more physical activity in at work. You might select from various channels available in your work site to conduct your physical activity program. Here are some ideas to target these employees.

What channels might you use to get your message to these employees?

- Conduct a lunch-time workshop on making time for physical activity or strategies for building in activity routinely throughout the day.
- Start an e-mail-based program that offers a tip of the day and provides encouragement and support through brief e-mailed feedback of employees' reported physical activity.
- Post energy expenditure charts.
- Conduct a lunchtime workshop on priority setting for exercise.
- Distribute print materials targeted toward individuals who are thinking about becoming more physically active.

What strategies might help these employees increase their physical activity?

- Encourage these employees to keep track of how much activity they are doing each week. Create a point system for making progress toward a physically active lifestyle. Make points redeemable for meaningful rewards such as donated gifts from local sponsors (USDHHS et al., 1999).
- Post cues by the elevator to take the stairs instead of the elevator.
- Help to set up informal physical activity support networks among the employees (USDHHS et al., 1999).
- Provide exercise prescriptions appropriate to employees' levels of fitness.
- Have employees monitor the minutes they spend sitting and being active during a day. Encourage them to replace sitting time with activity time.
- Encourage employees to hold one-on-one meetings while walking.
- Suggest that employees set their computer so it beeps as a reminder to take a 2-minute walk once each hour.

(continued)

(continued)

- Encourage employees to set a realistic goal for increasing the amount of activity they are doing.
- Provide opportunities for employees to practice new physical activity skills in a safe, non-judgmental environment.

What is an example of a special event that would be appropriate for employees in this stage?

- Plan an event called "Conquering Mount Everest" (Glaros, 1997).

  To prepare for this journey, a few calculations are necessary. The total height of Mount Everest is 29,028 feet. The distance between floors in most office buildings is 13 feet. One way to set up this journey is to have participants climb upward 130 feet per day (10 floors) five days per week. "Trek teams" with four members each would need approximately 11 weeks to complete the event.

  One person should be designated as the "Sherpa" to serve as team organizer and leader. Team members report their climbing success each week to the Sherpa who totals it and reports it to you.

  Alternatively, a drop box can be placed at the bottom of each stairwell with simple forms available for logging progress.

  Encourage your employees to add stair climbing to their daily routines rather than trying to do a week's worth of climbing in one day.

STAGE 4

Doing Enough Physical Activity

This group of employees has recently become active at the level recommended by national guidelines. Your program objective for this group will be to promote continued participation in activity for the long-term. To accomplish this you can do some of the following.

What channels might you use to get your message to these employees?

- Distribute print materials targeted toward individuals who are regularly physically active but only recently so.
- Set up a chat room on the intranet for problem solving.
- Conduct a lunchtime workshop on preventing boredom with physical activity.
- Start an e-mail-based program that offers a tip of the day and provides encouragement and support through brief e-mailed feedback of employees' reported physical activity.

What strategies might help these employees keep up their physical activity?

- Teach skills in alternative activities (in-line skating, tennis, kick-boxing, tae bo).
- Encourage employees to come up with a plan for maintaining and/or resuming physical activity during times when work and/or life is especially hectic.
- Sponsor an event that includes family and friends.
- Post mile markers on work-site grounds or measure the distance of inside routes (USDHHS et al., 1999).
- Negotiate deals for employees to use local exercise facilities.
- Give employees points for time spent being physically active each week and make points redeemable for small gift items such as exercise clothing, movie tickets, or passes to local exercise facilities or dances (USDHHS et al., 1999).

What further activities would be appropriate for employees in this stage?

- Encourage support groups (Glaros, 1997).

  Establish the need through surveys and focus groups.

  Create a mailing list for targeted individuals that you have discovered through any appropriate means. Provide employees on your list with supportive messages.

(continued)

(continued)

Publicize the group and establish an initial meeting time, date, and place.

Arrange for a content expert to be present at the initial meeting (who may also be available at future meetings on an as-needed basis). At the meeting, introduce your expert, determine the goals of the group, and share your own ideas for the group.

Identify potential group leaders who can assist in communications and logistics. Establish a proposed meeting schedule and use your connections to reserve rooms and obtain management permission if needed.

Attend occasional meetings yourself to keep in touch with their activities and status.

STAGE 5

Making Physical Activity a Habit

Employees in this stage are familiar with physical activity as they have been regularly active for at least six months. Your program objective will be to help them keep active by anticipating lapses, planning for situations that jeopardize their activity, and keeping them motivated over the long-term. Here are some suggestions for achieving these goals.

What strategies might help these employees prevent set-backs in their physical activity?

- Distribute print materials targeted toward individuals who are active and have been so for at least six months.
- Sponsor a charity walk/run.
- Give away pedometers or self-monitoring booklets or magnets with a self-monitoring form to encourage continued goal setting (see chapter 7).
- Ask these employees to sponsor a friend, family member, or co-worker who is trying to get started with physical activity.
- Give a workshop on injury prevention.
- Teach skills in alternative activities to decrease boredom.

What is an example of a special event that would be appropriate for employees in this stage?

- Celebrate National Jogging Day, which takes place in October and is an opportunity to either end the primary running season, or, especially in northern regions, prepare and encourage participants to continue running through the difficult winter months (Glaros, 1997).
- Organize a 10K/2K fun walk or run. Consider including family members for team events (for example, father and son) (Glaros, 1997).
- Begin a walking or running program with a destination-based or distance goal that culminates on either Thanksgiving or New Year's Day (Glaros, 1997).
- If your workplace is located in an area where the climate changes, host a seminar on performing physical activity in cold weather featuring both training methods and specialized clothing.
- Use the occasion to introduce running to interested non-runners.
- Organize a series of events featuring motorized treadmills as an alternative to outdoor winter walking or running.
- Promote active participation in your walking club, especially for new members.
- Develop a list of locations such as local colleges and community sports facilities that are suitable for indoor physical activity during the winter months. If possible, provide maps of locations (Glaros, 1997).

CONCLUSION

Many Americans work outside the home, so work-site physical activity programs have the potential to reach a lot of people. Traditional work-site programs have tended to attract only the employees most motivated for physical activity. However, a stage-matched approach, as described in this chapter, can attract and retain greater numbers of employees than traditional programs. We hope that this chapter has provided you with some useful ideas for developing and implementing a physical activity program that meets the needs of all the employees at your work site.

References

Dishman, R.K., Oldenburg, B., O'Neal, H., & Shephard, R.J. (1998). Worksite physical activity interventions. *American Journal of Preventive Medicine, 15,* 344–361.

Glaros, T.E. (1997). *Health promotion ideas that work: 84 proven activities for the workplace.* Champaign, IL: Human Kinetics.

Marcus, B.H., Emmons, K.M., Simkin-Silverman, L.R., Linnan, L.A., Taylor, E.R., Bock, B.C., et al. (1998). Evaluation of stage-matched versus standard self-help physical activity interventions at the workplace. *American Journal of Health Promotion, 12,* 246–253.

Sharratt, M.T., & Cox, M. (1988). Employee fitness: State of the art. *Canadian Journal of Public Health, 79,* S40–S43.

Shephard, R.J. (1992). A critical analysis of work-site fitness programs and their postulated economic benefits. *Medicine and Science in Sports and Exercise, 24,* 354–370.

U.S. Department of Health and Human Services. (1993). *1992 national survey of worksite health promotion activities.* Washington, DC: U.S. Government Printing Office.

U.S. Department of Health and Human Services, Public Health Service, Centers for Disease Control and Prevention, National Center for Chronic Disease Prevention and Health Promotion, & Division of Nutrition and Physical Activity. (1999). *Promoting physical activity: A guide for community action.* Champaign, IL: Human Kinetics

Wanzel, R.S. (1994). Decades of worksite fitness programmes: Progress or rhetoric? *Sports Medicine, 17,* 324–337.

ELEVEN

Using the Stages Model in Community Programs

By designing and implementing a community-based physical activity program, you can make an impact on the public health of your community, but developing a physical activity program to meet the needs of an entire community can be a daunting task. The individuals within any given community are sure to differ significantly, so whom should you target? What type of program can help these individuals the most? It also may be expensive to implement such a large-scale project. However, community programs have the potential to reach a great number of underactive individuals through various channels, such as mass media coverage, print materials, the inclusion of community leaders, and organized events like fun runs and health fairs. You can also reach a larger number of people in the community at a low cost per person by taking advantage of technologies such as the telephone, interactive computer systems, and the Internet (Marcus, Owen, Forsyth, Cavill, & Fridinger, 1998).

Community campaigns to improve cardiovascular risk factors including physical activity have been around for over three decades. Traditionally, programs such as the Stanford Five-City Project (Young, Haskel, Taylor, & Fortman, 1996) and the Minnesota Heart Health Program (Luepker, Murray, Jacobs, & Mittelmark, 1994) have targeted several cardiovascular risk factors, including high blood pressure, poor diet, and tobacco use, along with physical activity. They also tended to use a "one-size-fits-all" approach, in which a general message promoting physical activity was given to all individuals, regardless of their level of motivational readiness for taking up physical activity. While programs such as these helped increase awareness concerning physical activity, they were less effective at increasing physical activity behavior (Marcus, Owen, et al., 1998).

We have since learned that it is important to divide the population into subgroups (i.e., target audiences) and customize programs for each of these segments to better meet the needs of individuals within a community. Studies that have divided populations by motivational stage of readiness and then delivered stage-targeted messages have proven to be more successful than traditional approaches for getting people to change their behavior (Marcus, Bock, Pinto, Forsyth, Roberts, & Traficante, 1998; Marcus, Emmons et al., 1998). Chapter 6 provides a more detailed description of some of these programs, such as Jump Start to Health: A Workplace-Based Study and Jump Start: A Community-Based Study.

In this chapter we discuss how you can use the stages of motivational readiness to design a physical activity program for the people in your community and strategies that might be effective for these individuals. You can also refer to *Promoting Physical Activity: A Guide for Community Action* (USDHHS et al., 1999), which is an excellent resource for designing and implementing a community program. To begin, we discuss reasons to use the stages of motivational readiness to build your program.

Community Stage of Change

Traditionally, the stages of motivational readiness model is used to describe behavior change at the *individual* level (USDHHS et al., 1999). However, some have also applied it to entire communities to describe how ready a given community is to make physical activity a priority for its residents (Abrams, 1991; McLeroy, Bibeau, Steckler, & Glanz 1998; USDHHS et al., 1999). Researchers and health promoters alike have noted that environmental factors are important considerations for individual behavior change. For example, some environmental factors, such as building more bike and walking paths, enhance the likelihood of individual behavior change. Other variables, such as institutional factors, like an employer who does not give employees release time for physical activity, impede individual change. Societal factors within a community (e.g., support from community officials) also influence stages of physical activity readiness at a community level. As illustrated in figure 11.1, environmental, social, and institutional factors influence each other and are all important considerations in a community's stage of change. Here are other specific examples of how the stages of change can be interpreted at a community level (USDHHS et al., 1999, p. 62):

- A work site that is considering a change in employee health benefits to include physical activity incentives might be in stage 2, thinking about change.
- A work site whose administration is already taking the appropriate steps to institutionalize a cost-effective physical activity program might be in stage 5, making activity a habit.
- A school district that is piloting a model physical activity program in one of its schools may be in stage 3, doing some physical activity before adopting the program districtwide.
- A community in the construction phase of converting old railroad lines into pedestrian and bicycle pathways has demonstrated

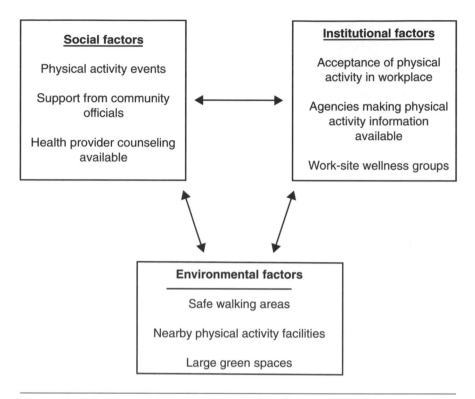

Figure 11.1 Influence of social, institutional, and environmental factors on community stage of change.

a commitment to physical activity and could be considered to be in stage 4, doing enough physical activity.

Determining the stage of motivational readiness of a community helps you learn the barriers to change at the community level (e.g., unsafe neighborhoods for walking, few activity-related events, lack of support by community officials) and the potential community supports for physical activity (e.g., health care providers willing to counsel their patients on physical activity, work-site wellness groups already in place). The community's motivational readiness for physical activity promotion can be determined in different ways. You might examine the community's physical environment, or you might conduct interviews with several community members of various characteristics to see whether they feel that the needed community support (e.g., safe walking areas, acceptance of physical activity in the workplace, nearby community exercise facilities) is in place for them to become or stay physically activity. You also should determine the community's commitment to physical-activity-related goals or practices (e.g., Are agencies willing to make physical activity information available? Are activity-related events taking place?). Your stage assessment should include the community's status on physical activity promoting actions, their intention to move toward them, and the steps they have taken or the plan they have in place for implementing them (USDHHS et al., 1999).

To determine the stage of motivational readiness at the community level, you need to assess a community's intention to change as well as its ability to achieve specific behavioral goals related to physical activity (USDHHS et al., 1999). Such behavioral goals might include the following actions in these areas:

- **Social networks:** Develop community walking groups. Foster collaborations among local health agencies. Encourage partnerships between businesses and exercise facilities. Generate a hotline to offer ideas, information, and encouragement to members of the community.
- **Environment:** Raise funds for more bike and walking paths. Build housing developments near exercise facilities. Promote public transportation. Install better lighting for sidewalks.
- **Community norms:** Encourage biking with helmets as a way to travel to work. Publicize the need for child care in fitness facilities. Have community leaders deliver physical activity messages.
- **Policies and legislation:** Lobby for tax cuts for work sites that promote physical activity for their employees. Pass zoning laws for green space.

Once you have determined the community's stage of motivational readiness for various program ideas that you have in mind, you can begin to think about how to meet the needs of individuals within the community.

Reaching Individuals Within a Community

It is an unrealistic goal to influence everyone in a given community. A more appropriate goal for a community physical activity program is to try to reach a majority of individuals within the community. Moreover, a program that tries to meet the needs of everyone within a community actually serves no one very well. As mentioned earlier, a general program does not account for individual differences that affect physical activity adoption. To make a program work for a large number of people, it is important to assess the needs of the people you are trying to reach (USDHHS et al., 1999). You can determine the stages of most people in the community and make a decision about your target audience that way, or you can choose your target audience and then determine the stages of the people within it. Before designing your program, find out what your target audience thinks about physical activity, why they might want to become more active, what has been holding them back, where they go to get their information, possible sources of support, and so on. You can then customize your message to meet the needs of your target audience. This plan is based on business marketing principles called *social marketing* (Kotler & Zaltman, 1971). Social marketing is an approach in which the marketer listens to what the consumer feels is best for him and formulates the solution to suit the consumer's perceptions rather than trying to tell a consumer what is best for him. Consumers' perceptions can be obtained through focus groups and personal interviews with representative people from the selected audience.

An example of the social-marketing approach is the Community Health Assessment and Promotion Project (CHAPP), a community nutrition and exercise program developed by the Emory University Department of Community Health and the Centers for Disease Control and targeted at overweight, inner-city, low-income African-American women in Atlanta, Georgia (Lasco, Curry, Dickson, Powers, Menes, & Merritt, 1989). While some health promoters feel that promoting physical activity for the poor or underprivileged is counterproductive because these individuals have more serious issues that require their attention, the CHAPP developers found that their target audience was actually quite interested in improving their health through better eating and physical activity. Participants in the CHAPP program reported that physical activity was an issue over which they were able to exert some control and becoming more active helped them to feel more empowered.

However, to make the program work in this urban community, the program developers found that it was important to ask participants to comment on the program during personal interviews and to incorporate their suggestions. For instance, the program planners learned that participants needed safe and comfortable ways to get to their activity. They accomplished this by providing security escorts for walking groups in dangerous neighborhoods. It was revealed that many of the participants felt uncomfortable performing exercise in front of people outside the program, so privacy blinds were installed in the aerobics classroom. The CHAPP program also arranged low-cost transportation and child care to remove some additional barriers. This example illustrates that by narrowing your focus to a particular group and asking them what they want in a program, you can include elements that better fit their needs.

Developing Stage-Matched Messages

Targeted and *tailored* physical activity messages are two strategies based on social-marketing principles (figure 11.2). A targeted program involves defining groups within the population along some characteristic, such as stage of motivational readiness, and then delivering a program suited to this characteristic. A targeted approach assumes that the members of a defined group are similar enough for one message to effectively communicate to all members of the group. Targeting by stage of motivational readiness and then delivering stage-matched printed materials about physical activity has been shown to effectively increase physical

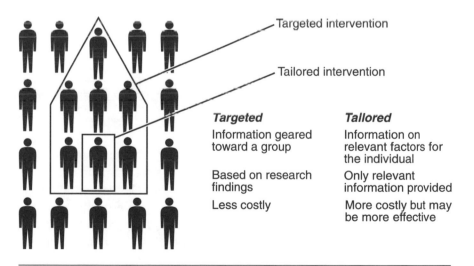

Targeted intervention

Tailored intervention

Targeted	**Tailored**
Information geared toward a group	Information on relevant factors for the individual
Based on research findings	Only relevant information provided
Less costly	More costly but may be more effective

Figure 11.2   Targeted vs. tailored approaches to physical activity promotion.

activity behavior (Marcus, Banspach, Lefebvre, Rossi, Carleton, & Abrams, 1992; Marcus, Emmons, et al., 1998). Chapter 6 provides more detailed descriptions of these programs, such as Imagine Action and Jump Start to Health: A Workplace-Based Study.

A *tailored* program is customized to each member of a specified stage. Each person answers questions about factors important to changing her behavior (e.g., her level of confidence in being physically active, her use of relevant cognitive and behavioral strategies, her outcome expectations). Then each person's answers are used to create messages that are personally relevant (Marcus, Nigg, Riebe, & Forsyth, 2000). Although the tailored approach needs more testing, we believe that providing people with personally relevant messages will increase the likelihood that they read and process the message. This in turn should increase the likelihood that they use the information to change behavior.

While providing an individually tailored, stage-matched message about physical activity sounds ideal, it is more expensive and labor intensive to tailor a message than it is to deliver a targeted one. You need to weigh the costs and benefits of each when you select between a targeted or tailored approach. However, in some cases, technologies such as computers and the Internet can be used to individually tailor physical activity messages in a cost-effective manner. Moreover, technologies such as these allow us to move beyond reliance on face-to-face counseling to affordable, individually tailored counseling on a large scale (Marcus, Bock, et al., 1998; see chapter 6 for a description of a program that used computer-generated tailored messages, such as Jump Start: A Community-Based Study).

Using a Media-Based Approach to Reach Your Target Audience

A recent review of 127 published physical activity studies from the years 1965 through 1995 found that interventions using a media-based approach to deliver programs (e.g., print mailings, telecommunications) were more effective than programs that were delivered face to face (Dishman & Buckworth, 1996). Media-based approaches may be more effective because they allow individuals more flexibility and choice in how they implement their physical activity programs, while face-to-face programs usually entail some type of physical activity done in the presence of the counselor. Moreover, we can reach most households by mail or telephone. Print-based, stage-targeted physical activity programs delivered to sedentary adults by mail have been found to successfully help them become more active (e.g., Cardinal & Sachs, 1996; Marcus et al., 1992), as have print-based, tailored, self-help physical activity programs (Marcus, Bock, et al., 1998). Participants can be mailed the stages-of-change questionnaire (see chapter 2) along with other relevant measures, such as self-efficacy, decisional balance, and processes-of-change questionnaires (see chapter 5). They can then receive personally relevant printed materials within a day or two of mailing their questionnaires.

The telephone is another avenue for reaching large numbers of individuals within a community. Around 95 percent of Americans have a telephone in their homes (Fowler, 1993; Lavrakas, 1987; table 11.1). Physical activity counseling by telephone helps sedentary people become more active. For example, a study in which health educators with bachelor's degrees counseled sedentary older adults about home-based physical activity found that telephone counseling led to better adherence to moderate- and vigorous-intensity physical activity than a structured exercise class did (King, Taylor, Haskell, & DeBusk, 1988; King, Haskell, Taylor, Kraemar, & DeBusk, 1991).

Another study is underway that is comparing the effectiveness of physical activity counseling provided via telephone by a health educator versus a computer that people access by telephone (King et al., in press). In the computer-based program, participants use the touch pad on their telephone to enter in their weekly minutes of activity or their intention to become active, their activity goals for the upcoming week, and whether or not they would like to hear information on relevant topics regarding physical activity. The computer system stores their data and delivers recorded voice messages that are appropriate for their stage

Table 11.1 Computer and Internet Access in U.S. Homes

	1984	1989	1993	1997	1998	2000
% with telephone	91.8	93.0	94.2	90.9	94.1	94.8
% with computer	8.2	15.0	22.8	36.6	42.1	51.0
% with Internet	*	*	*	18.0	26.2	41.5

Note: Data on internet access were not collected before 1997.

From US Census Bureau, Current Population Survey.

of motivational readiness. Telephone programs such as these have the advantage of providing on-the-spot support and feedback (Marcus et al., 2000), and they have been shown to be effective in previous studies (Pinto, Friedman, Marcus, Lin, Fennstedt, & Gillman, 2000). They also can be used proactively to dial out to individuals rather than waiting for individuals to call in to the system. Moreover, people can also call in for physical activity counseling when they feel the need, regardless of the time of day or the day of the week (Marcus et al., 2000). The ability to receive physical activity counseling at any time when needed is usually not an option when a real person delivers the counseling.

There has been a dramatic increase in the percentage of U.S. households with personal computers: from 8 percent in 1984 to 45 percent in 1998 (U.S. Bureau of the Census, n.d.; see table 11.1). As of 1998, there were more than 70 million U.S. adults actively using the Internet (Nielsen Media Research, 1998; Wiese, 1999), with one half using the Internet to obtain health information (FIND/SVP, 1997). Programs are currently underway in which the participants fill out stages-of-change questions on a Web site and are then given stage-relevant messages and links to other relevant stage-appropriate Web sites. Using the World Wide Web to deliver the program allows participants to get the types of information in which they are interested and also teaches them to gather information for themselves. E-mail and online chat boards are avenues for providing support and encouragement from program leaders and other program participants, again, at any time of the day or night so that whenever a person is experiencing a barrier or dealing with a lapse, help is available. Technologies such as the Internet and computerized telephone systems are not only more cost effective than face-to-face programs, they also provide the community with better access and availability to physical activity advice.

Working With Community Leaders to Reach Your Target Audience

Another promising method for delivering community physical activity programs is taking advantage of the individuals who have the greatest influence over the groups of people you are trying to reach (King, 1998). These influential people might include physicians, reporters, journalists, and teachers. For example, you can develop a course about physical activity promotion that offers continuing education credits to train physicians, nurses, psychologists, and other health professionals to deliver stage-matched physical activity counseling to their patients (King, 1998). Similarly, you can offer training to physical education instructors in promoting lifestyle activity among their students by encouraging them to use relevant cognitive and behavioral strategies (King, 1998).

Politicians, members of the clergy, and other community leaders also influence public opinion and can be helpful by endorsing your program to the community or at least to their constituents in the community you are targeting. The impetus for the CHAPP program described earlier came from the members of the targeted community itself who formed a coalition that studied the needs of their community and designed a program accordingly. The coalition worked together with the program developers to design a program that had low attrition rates and produced clinically significant reductions in weight and blood pressure in the targeted group of overweight, inner-city African-American women, a group that often has high attrition rates in health promotion programs (Lasco et al., 1989).

Stage-Specific Strategies for Community Physical Activity Programs

We created the following list of intervention strategies to help you design your own community program. As we have tried to stress in this and other chapters, no one program works for everyone so we do not provide a step-by-step program development guide. Rather, we hope that you might pick some of the following strategies plus generate some of your own ideas so that you create a program that meets the needs of your target audience, your community's stage of change, any time constraints you may be working under, and your financial resources.

STAGE 1

Not Thinking About Change

For this segment of the population, your goal is to help increase awareness about the (a) benefits of physical activity, (b) support for it in the local community, and (c) acceptance of physical activity by other community members. Here are some strategies for increasing awareness and encouraging people to begin to think about the role physical activity could play in their lives.

What communication channels might you use to reach people not considering becoming active?

- Distribute print materials targeted toward individuals who are presently not thinking about becoming more physically active.

- Work with the media to gain visibility for your messages. You might achieve this by doing the following (USDHHS et al., 1999):

  Invite newspaper reporters to visible or newsworthy events.

  Work with reporters in writing feature stories.

  Provide timely news releases or newspaper articles.

  Participate as a guest on radio or television talk shows.

  Purchase radio, television, or cable advertising time.

- Display key messages and your program logo in storefront windows or community bulletin boards, on billboard signs, and as banners across the main street or at major community locations (USDHHS et al., 1999).

- Design bumper stickers with physical activity and health promotion messages (USDHHS et al., 1999).

- Ask utility companies, banks, physicians, and others to place promotional and educational information in their monthly billings. Ask to place promotional and educational materials in waiting rooms of hospitals and health maintenance organizations, private physician offices, clinics, mental health centers, and senior citizen centers (USDHHS et al., 1999).

What types of information are most relevant to individuals in this earliest stage?

- Host health fairs that include exercise testing, blood pressure screenings, or body fat composition assessments. Relate how these are affected by physical activity.

- Emphasize the short-term benefits of being active (e.g., feeling invigorated, sleeping better, reducing stress, feeling better about oneself) rather than the long-term benefits that these individuals might feel are unobtainable.

- Dispel possible misconceptions about physical activity (e.g., "No pain, no gain," overestimated risk of injuries such as heart attack).
- Increase awareness of what they might miss by choosing not to be active (e.g., enjoyment from being active, better self-esteem).

What are some other strategies that might move these individuals closer to considering change?

- Help people to visualize success—to visualize a happy, healthy and active lifestyle.
- Encourage these individuals to read or think about how physical activity might benefit them. For this group, it is better to focus on the benefits of physical activity and not to dwell on the risks of a sedentary lifestyle.
- Link benefits of a physically active lifestyle to people's highest priorities and values in life (e.g., relationship with family, personal faith, health, or happiness).
- Encourage these individuals to see how their sedentary behavior affects them personally and others in their life (e.g., a sedentary parent models an unhealthy lifestyle to her children).

How might you show community support for physical activity?

- Work with health care providers to encourage them to advise their patients on how they might benefit from physical activity.
- Choose a spokesperson that the target audience trusts, respects, believes, or can identify with to help increase awareness. Identify role models within the community. Recruit local people to endorse your program (USDHHS et al., 1999).
- Conduct targeted informational campaigns and sessions (USDHHS et al., 1999):

  Lunch-n-learn or community lectures

  Workshops, seminars, or adult education classes

  Youth group programs

  One-on-one counseling or instruction

  Guest talk-show appearances on television and radio

  Columns or featured articles in the newspaper
- Give informative presentations to work sites, schools, and community organizations, such as Rotary Clubs, Business and Professional Women, or the American Association of Retired Persons (USDHHS et al., 1999).

STAGE 2

Thinking About Change

For this segment of the community, one of your goals is to help increase awareness of the benefits of physical activity, community support, and the social norms for this behavior. The second goal is to move these individuals closer to actually trying out the behavior. Here are some ideas for achieving these goals.

What communication channels might you use?

- Distribute print materials targeted toward individuals who are thinking about becoming more physically active or include health and physical activity tips in general publications (USDHHS et al., 1999).

- Increase awareness by working with the media to gain visibility for your messages (USDHHS et al., 1999):

  Invite newspaper reporters to visible or newsworthy events.

  Work with reporters in writing feature stories.

  Provide timely news releases or newspaper articles.

  Participate as a guest on radio or television talk shows.

  Purchase radio, television, or cable advertising time.

- Display key messages and your program logo in storefront windows or community bulletin boards, on billboard signs, and as banners across the main street or at major community locations (USDHHS et al., 1999).

- Design bumper stickers with physical activity and health promotion messages.

- Ask utility companies, banks, physicians, and others to place promotional and educational information in their monthly billings. Ask to place promotional and educational materials in waiting rooms of hospitals and health maintenance organizations, private physician offices, clinics, mental health centers, and senior citizen centers (USDHHS et al., 1999).

- Make health videos available at video stores and libraries.

- Set up a Web site with links to relevant stage-appropriate physical activity and health sites.

What types of information are most relevant to individuals who are considering becoming more active?

- Provide basic information needed to achieve a physically active lifestyle such as selecting the appropriate shoes or clothing (USDHHS et al., 1999).

- Describe a variety of activities available to most people that can be done alone or with family and friends.

- Suggest ways to build in some activity into one's daily routine (e.g., taking the stairs at work).
- Dispel possible misconceptions about physical activity (e.g., "No pain, no gain," overestimated risk of injury such as heart attack).

What are some other strategies that might move these individuals closer to trying some physical activity?

- Provide messages that link physical activity to values or issues relevant to your target audience.
- Help them weigh the pros and cons of a physically active lifestyle. Focus on the costs of changing (effort, energy, and the things they must give up to overcome a sedentary lifestyle) and how they might deal with them.
- Encourage them to start off slowly (e.g., 5- or 10-minute walk) and build gradually (add 5 minutes per day per week) and how to reward their achievement of these goals.
- Give out self-assessment questionnaires such as the Physical Activity Readiness Questionnaire (PAR-Q, found in chapter 8) and the Decisional Balance Questionnaire (found in chapter 5).
- Help people to visualize success—to visualize a happy, healthy, and active lifestyle.

How might you show community support for beginning to try some physical activity?

- Host health fairs that include exercise testing, blood pressure screenings, or body fat composition assessments. Relate how these are affected by physical activity.
- Choose a spokesperson that the target audience trusts, respects, believes, or can identify with. Identify role models within the community. Recruit local people to endorse your program (USDHHS et al., 1999).
- Work with health care providers and encourage them to advise these patients on how they might benefit from physical activity and some steps they could take to begin a physically active lifestyle.
- Conduct targeted informational campaigns and sessions through (USDHHS et al., 1999):

  Lunch-n-learn or community lectures

  Workshops, seminars, or adult education classes

  Youth group programs

  One-on-one counseling or instruction

(continued)

197

(continued)

Guest talk-show appearances on television and radio

Columns or featured articles in the newspaper

- Give informative presentations to work sites, schools, and community organizations, such as Rotary Clubs, Business and Professional Women, or the American Association of Retired Persons (USDHHS et al., 1999).
- Set-up physical activity "hotlines" so that people can call with questions on physical activity (USDHHS et al., 1999).

STAGE 3

Doing Some Physical Activity

Individuals in this stage are likely to be receptive to physical activity messages, since they are doing some activity but not enough to meet national guidelines. Therefore, your goal for this group is to encourage them to increase the amount of physical activity they do each week. To accomplish this goal you might choose to do some of the following.

What communication channels might you use to reach these individuals?

- Distribute print materials targeted toward individuals who want to become more physically active.
- Develop or make available self-instructional materials, such as videotaped instruction, cassette tape instruction, computer-based instruction, how-to guides, manuals, and kits (USDHHS et al., 1999).
- Provide formal and informal activity-oriented instructional programs, such as workshops, classes, seminars, demonstrations, lessons, and lectures (USDHHS et al., 1999).
- Sponsor "meet the expert" events so community members can learn directly from those who have mastered various skills (USDHHS et al., 1999).
- Set up "hotlines" so that people can call with questions on physical activity (USDHHS et al., 1999).
- Set up a Web site with links to relevant physical activity and health sites.

What types of information are most relevant to individuals who need to increase their level of physical activity?

- Discuss how to develop a plan for regular activity.
- Provide ideas for making activity more fun.
- Teach methods for self-monitoring for keeping track of progress.
- Discuss barriers and ways to overcome them.
- Suggest ways the reader might restructure her environment to make it more probable she will be active and less likely to be sedentary (e.g., move exercise equipment where she will see it rather than hiding it in the basement; keep walking shoes at work or by the door at home).
- Discuss ways to use exercise or sports equipment properly and safely.
- Describe stretching, warm-up, and cool-down techniques.

(continued)

199

(continued)

What are some other strategies that might move these individuals closer to meeting national guidelines for regular activity?

- Host health and fitness fairs that include exercise testing to demonstrate that each person needs more physical activity (USDHHS et al., 1999).
- Emphasize small, specific, and realistic goals.
- Encourage use of self-rewards for meeting goals.
- Encourage the reader to make use of social support networks such as walking clubs or friends or co-workers who exercise during lunch breaks.
- Suggest exercising while sitting in a chair, standing, or watching television.
- Start a walking or jogging program.

How might you show community support for increasing physical activity?

- Develop a community resource list so that people will know where to find courses or opportunities to develop skills.
- Appeal to the community's competitive spirit with contests, prizes, incentives, publicity, recognition, rewards, and fun promotional items. Establish competitive programs between individuals, neighborhoods, churches, organizations, or businesses. Incentives might include discounts for recreational facilities, fitness club memberships, sports or exercise equipment or apparel, a free lunch, book, T-shirt, or pair of walking shoes, public recognition, community awards, and so on (USDHHS et al., 1999).
- Work with health care providers to encourage them to advise their patients to increase their levels of physical activity and to take advantage of the many community resources you can identify.
- Provide opportunities to try different types of physical activity for just one day or for one event (USDHHS et al., 1999):
  Community walking events
  Using stairs instead of elevators for one day or one week
  Bicycle-to-work day or other bicycling events
  Periodic fun-runs
  Lunchtime walking groups at local businesses, schools, or shopping malls
  Trial memberships and guest passes to use recreational facilities
- For groups of various ages or levels of experience, work with physical education instructors, physical therapists, or exercise physiologists to design appropriate and quality instructional programs.

Doing Enough Physical Activity

This is a group of individuals who have recently become active at the level recommended by national guidelines. Your goal is to foster continued participation in physical activity and to bolster continued community support for activity. To accomplish this you can do some of the following.

What communication channels might you use to reach regularly active individuals?

- Distribute print materials targeted toward individuals who are physically active at the level recommended by national guidelines but at risk for relapse.
- Set-up telephone "hotlines" so that people can call with questions on physical activity (USDHHS et al., 1999).
- Develop a community resource list so that people will know where to find courses or opportunities to develop new skills.
- Sponsor "meet the expert" events so that community members can learn directly from those who have mastered various skills (USDHHS et al., 1999).
- Set up a Web site with links to relevant physical activity and health sites.

What types of information are most relevant to individuals who are regularly active?

- Provide a list of activities that will reduce the risk of injury and boredom and encourage trying different activities.
- Describe stretching, warm-up, and cool-down techniques.
- Suggest ways to restructure one's environment (e.g., move exercise equipment where she will see it rather than hiding it in the basement; keep walking shoes at work or by the door at home) to make it more probable that one chooses an active pursuit rather than a sedentary one.
- Instruct on how to avoid the risks of injury from exercise.
- Teach self-monitoring methods for keeping track of progress.

What are some other strategies to help these individuals stay active?

- Encourage use of social support networks such as walking clubs or friends or co-workers who exercise during lunch breaks.
- Instruct on how to anticipate lapses and accept them as a normal part of the change process so that the occasional lapse is not viewed as a failure.

(continued)

(continued)

- Help identify situations that are more likely to lead to a lapse and develop a plan for keeping active in these situations.
- Encourage these individuals to build in rewards to maintain motivation. These can be tangible such as a new pair of walking shoes or intangible such as taking a mental note of achieving a goal.
- Help these individuals develop long-range goals for physical activity (e.g., participating in a 5-mile fun-walk in a few months) and short-term goals to help reach the long-term goal (e.g., increasing the distance walked by 1/2 mile per week).

How might you show community support for staying physically active at nationally recommended levels?

- Appeal to the community's competitive spirit with contests, prizes, incentives, publicity, recognition, rewards, and fun promotional items. Establish competitive programs between individuals, neighborhoods, churches, organizations, or businesses. Incentives might include discounts for recreational facilities, fitness club memberships, sports or exercise equipment or apparel, a free lunch, book, T-shirt, or pair of walking shoes, public recognition, community awards, and so on (USDHHS et al., 1999).
- Work with health care providers to encourage them to ask their patients about physical activity and tell their patients about community resources for physical activity.
- Provide opportunities to try different types of physical activity for just one day or for one event (USDHHS et al., 1999):

  Community walking events

  Using stairs instead of elevators for one day or one week

  Bicycle-to-work day or other bicycling events

  Periodic fun-runs

  Lunchtime walking groups at local businesses, schools, or shopping malls

  Trial memberships and guest passes to use recreational facilities

STAGE 5

Making Physical Activity a Habit

This audience is one who is familiar with physical activity as they have been regularly active for at least six months. You goal is to help them keep active by anticipating lapses, planning for situations that jeopardize their activity, and keeping them motivated over the long-term. Here are some suggestions for achieving these goals.

What communication channels might you use to reach regularly active individuals?

- Distribute print materials targeted toward individuals who are active and have been so for at least six months.
- Provide a list of activities that will reduce the risk of injury and boredom and encourage the reader to try different activities.
- Set-up telephone "hotlines" so that people can call with questions on physical activity or activity related injuries (USDHHS et al., 1999).
- Develop a community resource list so that people will know where to find courses or opportunities to develop new activity skills.
- Sponsor "meet the expert" events so community members can learn directly from those who have mastered various skills that may be new to these individuals (USDHHS et al., 1999).

What types of information are most relevant to individuals in this stage?

- Teach how to anticipate lapses and accept them as a normal part of the change process so that the occasional lapse is not viewed as a failure.
- Help identify situations more likely to lead to a lapse and how one might develop a plan for keeping active in these situations.
- Remind regularly active individuals to build in rewards to maintain motivation. These can be tangible such as a new pair of walking shoes or intangible such as making a mental note of achieving a goal.
- Provide a list of activities that will reduce the risk of injury and boredom and encourage trying different activities.

What are some other strategies to help these individuals stay active?

- Encourage use of social support networks such as walking clubs or friends or co-workers who exercise during lunch breaks.
- Help the individual recognize and appreciate her personal responsibility for successfully maintaining change.
- Give suggestions for how the individual might serve as a role model for others.

(continued)

(continued)

How might you show community support for maintenance of regular physical activity?

- Appeal to the community's competitive spirit with contests, prizes, incentives, publicity, recognition, rewards, and fun promotional items. Establish competitive programs between individuals, neighborhoods, churches, organizations, or businesses. Incentives might include discounts for recreational facilities, fitness club memberships, sports or exercise equipment or apparel, a free lunch, book, T-shirt, or pair of walking shoes, public recognition, community awards, and so on (USDHHS et al., 1999).

- Work with health care providers and encourage them to ask their patients about physical activity and counsel on relapse prevention.

- Provide opportunities to try different types of physical activity for just one day or for one event (USDHHS et al., 1999):

  Community walking events

  Using stairs instead of elevators for one day or one week

  Bicycle-to-work day or other bicycling events

  Periodic fun-runs

  Lunchtime walking groups at local businesses, schools, or shopping malls

  Trial memberships and guest passes to use recreational facilities

CONCLUSION

Once you have determined who you want to target in your community program, what that group's needs and perceptions about physical activity are, the types of messages you want to deliver, and the means by which you will deliver your program, it is time to put your program together. The strategies you select are based on the scale of your project and the funds available. The Stage-Specific Strategies section offers some suggestions for print materials, media coverage, and community events based on your target audience's motivational readiness for changing their physical activity behavior. You can use these and your own ideas to improve physical activity participation in your community.

References

Abrams, D.B. (1991). Conceptual models to integrate individual and public health interventions: The example of the workplace. In *Proceedings of the International Conference on Promoting Dietary Change in Communities* (pp. 170–190). Seattle: Fred Hutchinson Cancer Research Center.

Cardinal, B.J., & Sachs, M.L. (1996). Effects of mail-mediated, stage-matched exercise behavior change strategies on female adults' leisure-time exercise behavior. *Journal of Sports Medicine and Physical Fitness, 36,* 100–107.

Dishman, R.K., & Buckworth, J. (1996). Increasing physical activity: A quantitative synthesis. *Medicine and Science in Sports and Exercise, 28,* 706–719.

FIND/SVP, Inc. (1997, May). *The 1997 American Internet user survey.* New York: Cyber Dialog, Inc.

Fowler, F.J., Jr. (1993). *Survey research methods* (2nd ed.). Newbury Park, CA: Sage.

King, A.C. (1998). How to promote physical activity in the community: Research experiences from the U.S. highlighting different community approaches. *Patient Education and Counseling, 33,* S3–S12.

King, A.C., Friedman, R., Marcus, B.H., Castro, C., Forsyth, L.H., Napolitano, M., et al. (in press). Harnessing motivational forces in the promotion of physical activity: The Community Health Advice by Telephone (CHAT) project. *Health Education Research,* special issue.

King, A.C., Haskell, W.L., Taylor, C.B., Kraemer, H.C., & DeBusk, R.F. (1991). Group vs. home-based exercise training in healthy older men and women. *Journal of the American Medical Association, 266,* 1535–1542.

King, A.C., Taylor, C.B., Haskell, W.L., & DeBusk, R.F. (1988). Strategies for increasing early adherence to and long-term maintenance of home-based exercise training in healthy middle-aged men and women. *American Journal of Cardiology, 61,* 628–632.

Kotler, P., & Zaltman, G. (1971). Social marketing: An approach to planned social change. *Journal of Marketing, 35,* 3–12.

Lasco, R.A., Curry, R.H., Dickson, V.J., Powers, J., Menes, S., & Merritt, R.K. (1989). Participation rates, weight loss, and blood pressure changes among obese women in a nutrition–exercise program. *Public Health Reports, 104,* 640–646.

Lavrakas, P.J. (1987). *Telephone survey methods: Sampling, selection, and supervision.* Newbury Park, CA: Sage.

Luepker, R.V., Murray, D.M., Jacobs, D.R., Jr., & Mittelmark, M.B. (1994). Community education for cardiovascular disease prevention: Risk factor changes in the Minnesota Heart Health Program. *American Journal of Public Health, 84,* 1383–1393.

Marcus, B.H., Banspach, S.W., Lefebvre, R.C., Rossi, J.S., Carleton, R.A., & Abrams, D.B. (1992). Using the stages of change model to increase the adoption of physical activity among community participants. *American Journal of Health Promotion, 6,* 424–429.

Marcus, B.H., Bock, B.C., Pinto, B.M., Forsyth, L.H., Roberts, M., & Traficante, R. (1998). Efficacy of individualized, motivationally tailored physical activity intervention. *Annals of Behavioral Medicine, 20,* 174–180.

Marcus, B.H., Emmons, K.M., Simkin-Silverman, L.R., Linnan, L.A., Taylor, E.R., Bock, B.C., et al. (1998). Evaluation of stage-matched versus standard self-help physical activity interventions at the workplace. *American Journal of Health Promotion, 12,* 246–253.

Marcus, B.H., Nigg, C.R., Riebe, D., & Forsyth, L.H. (2000). Interactive, preventive communication strategies: A proactive approach for reaching out to large populations. *American Journal of Health Promotion, 19*(2), 121–126.

Marcus, B.H., Owen, N., Forsyth, L.H., Cavill, N.A., & Fridinger, F. (1998). Physical activity interventions using mass media, print media, and information technology. *American Journal of Preventive Medicine, 15,* 362–378.

McLeroy, K.R., Bibeau, D., Steckler, A., & Glanz, K. (1998). An ecological perspective on health promotion programs. *Health Education Quarterly, 15,* 351–377.

Nielsen Media Research. (1998, August 24). *Number of Internet users and shoppers surges in United States and Canada.* New York: Author. Available: **www.nielsenmedia.com/newsreleases/releases/1998/commnet2.html**

Pinto, B.M., Friedman, R., Marcus, B.H., Lin, T., Fennstedt, S., & Gillman, M. (2000). Physical activity promotion using a computer-based telephone counseling system. *Annals of Behavioral Medicine, 22*(Suppl.), 212.

U.S. Bureau of the Census. (n.d.). *Level of access and use of computers: 1984, 1989, and 1993.* Washington, DC: Author. Available: **www.census.gov/population/socdemo/computer/report93/compusea.txt**

U.S. Department of Health and Human Services, Public Health Service, Centers for Disease Control and Prevention, National Center for Chronic Disease Prevention and Health Promotion, & Division of Nutrition and Physical Activity. (1999). *Promoting physical activity: A guide for community action.* Champaign, IL: Human Kinetics.

Wiese, E. (1999, January 26). America's online: 70.5 million adults. *USA Today Tech Report.* Available: **www.usatoday.com/life/cyber/tech/ctd392.htm**.

Young, D.R., Haskell, W.L., Taylor, C.B., & Fortmann, S.P. (1996). Effect of community health education on physical activity knowledge, attitudes, and behavior. *American Journal of Epidemiology, 144,* 264–274.

The following is a list of organizations and suggested readings you can use to enhance your programs.

Organizations

American Association for Active Lifestyles and Fitness (AAALF)
    1900 Association Drive
    Reston, VA 20191-1599
    800-213-7193
    http://www.aahperd.org/aaalf/aaalf/html

American College of Sports Medicine (ACSM)
    PO Box 1440
    Indianapolis, IN 46206-1440
    317-637-9200
    http://www.acsm.org/sportsmed

American Heart Association
    National Center
    7272 Greenville Avenue
    Dallas, TX 75231-4596
    214-373-6300
    http://www.americanheart.org

Centers for Disease Control and Prevention (CDC)
    National Center for Chronic Disease Prevention
        and Health Promotion
    Division of Nutrition and Physical Activity
    Mail Stop K-46
    4770 Buford Highway, NE
    Atlanta, GA 30341-3717
    770-488-5820
    http://www.cdc.gov/nccdphp/dnpa

The Cooper Institute for Aerobics Research
    12330 Preston Road
    Dallas, TX 75230
    972-341-3200 or 800-635-7050
    http://www.cooperinst.org

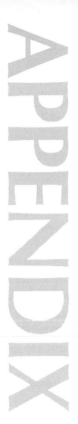

Human Kinetics
  PO Box 5076
  1607 N. Market Street
  Champaign, IL 61825-5076
  800-747-4457
  http://www.HumanKinetics.com

National Heart, Lung, and Blood Institute (NHLBI)
  National Institute of Health
  Building 31, Room 4A-21
  Bethesda, MD 20892
  301-251-1222
  http://www.nhlbi.nih.gov/nhlbi/nhlbi.htm

President's Council on Physical Fitness and Sports (PCPFS)
  200 Independence Avenue SW
  Huber H. Humphrey Bldg. Room 738H
  Washington, DC 20201-0004
  202-690-9000
  E-mail: cspain@osophs.dhhs.gov

Health Promotion Resource Center (HPRC)
  Stanford Center for Research in Disease Prevention
  730 Welch Road, Suite B
  Palo Alto, CA 94304
  650-723-0003

Centers for Behavioral and Preventive Medicine
  The Miriam Hospital
  Coro Building, Suite 5000
  1 Hoppin Street
  Providence, RI 02903
  401-793-8176
  Email: LSExercise@lifespan.org

Suggested Readings

A collection of physical activity questionnaires for health-related research. (1997). *Medicine and Science in Sports and Exercise, 29*(Suppl. 6).

American College of Sports Medicine. (1995). *Guidelines for exercise testing and prescription* (5th ed.). Baltimore: Williams & Wilkins.

Blair, S.N., Dunn, A.L., Marcus, B.H., Carpenter, R.A., & Jaret, P. (2001). *Active Living Every Day: 20 Weeks to Lifelong Vitality.* Champaign, IL: Human Kinetics.

Bouchard, C., Shephard, R., & Stephens, T. (1993). *Physical Activity, Fitness, and Health: International Proceedings and Consensus Statement.* Champaign, IL: Human Kinetics.

Centers for Disease Control. (1999). *Promoting Physical Activity: A Guide for Community Action.* Champaign, IL: Human Kinetics.

Glaros, T.E. (1997). *Health Promotion Ideas that Work: 84 Proven Activities for the Workplace.* Champaign, IL: Human Kinetics.

Marcus, B.H., Owen, N., Forsyth, L.H., Cavill, N.A. & Fridinger, F. (1998). Physical activity interventions using mass media, print media, and information technology. *American Journal of Preventive Medicine 15*(4), 362-378.

Measurement of physical activity [Special issue]. (2000). *Research Quarterly for Exercise and Sport, 71.*

U.S. Department of Health and Human Services. (1996). *Physical activity and health: A report of the Surgeon General.* Atlanta, GA: Centers for Disease Control and Prevention, National Center for Chronic Disease Prevention and Health Promotion.

Note: The italicized *f* and *t* following page numbers refer to figures and tables, respectively.

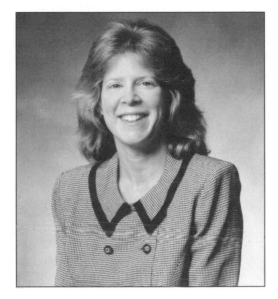

Bess H. Marcus, PhD, is a professor of psychiatry and human behavior at the Brown University Medical School. She is the director of physical activity research at the Brown University Center for Behavioral and Preventive Medicine at The Miriam Hospital. Dr. Marcus, a clinical and health psychologist, has spent the past 18 years conducting research on physical activity behavior, and she has published more than 100 papers and book chapters on this topic.

She has helped create new recommendations regarding the quantity and intensity of physical activity necessary for health benefits. She also contributed to the recent Surgeon General's Report on Physical Activity and Health. Dr. Marcus is known internationally for her work in helping people to become more physically active as she has spoken on this topic worldwide. She also served as an advisor on the curriculum development for Project Active and PRIME and is a coauthor of *Active Living Every Day*.

Dr. Marcus makes time to be physically active on most days of the week. She enjoys cycling, swimming, and walking with her husband, children, and friends.

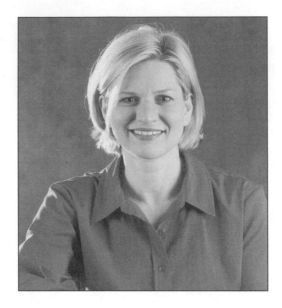

LeighAnn Forsyth, PhD, is an assistant professor of psychology at Cleveland State University where she conducts research on physical activity promotion and weight management. She serves as a consultant for several NIH-funded programs promoting physical activity in diverse populations. She has coauthored invited consensus documents on physical activity maintenance and the efficacy of mediated physical activity programs. Dr. Forsyth, a clinical and health psychologist, also has a private practice specializing in eating disorders, body image, and weight management. Dr. Forsyth completed a clinical internship and a two-year postdoctoral fellowship at the Brown University Center for Behavioral and Preventive Medicine at The Miriam Hospital. She also participated in several research programs applying the stages of motivational readiness to promote physical activity adoption. She enjoys walking, in-line skating, weight-lifting, and running after her two children.